Disorders of Motor, Somatic and Cognitive Development in Children with Neurodysfunctions

Disorders of Motor, Somatic and Cognitive Development in Children with Neurodysfunctions

Editors

Agnieszka Guzik
Lidia Perenc
Mariusz Drużbicki

MDPI • Basel • Beijing • Wuhan • Barcelona • Belgrade • Manchester • Tokyo • Cluj • Tianjin

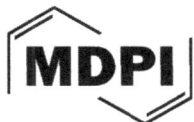

Editors
Agnieszka Guzik
University of Rzeszów
Poland

Lidia Perenc
University of Rzeszów
Poland

Mariusz Drużbicki
University of Rzeszów
Poland

Editorial Office
MDPI
St. Alban-Anlage 66
4052 Basel, Switzerland

This is a reprint of articles from the Special Issue published online in the open access journal *Children* (ISSN 2227-9067) (available at: https://www.mdpi.com/journal/children/special_issues/neurodysfunctions).

For citation purposes, cite each article independently as indicated on the article page online and as indicated below:

LastName, A.A.; LastName, B.B.; LastName, C.C. Article Title. *Journal Name* **Year**, *Volume Number*, Page Range.

ISBN 978-3-0365-0726-2 (Hbk)
ISBN 978-3-0365-0727-9 (PDF)

© 2021 by the authors. Articles in this book are Open Access and distributed under the Creative Commons Attribution (CC BY) license, which allows users to download, copy and build upon published articles, as long as the author and publisher are properly credited, which ensures maximum dissemination and a wider impact of our publications.

The book as a whole is distributed by MDPI under the terms and conditions of the Creative Commons license CC BY-NC-ND.

Contents

About the Editors vii

Preface to "Disorders of Motor, Somatic and Cognitive Development in Children with Neurodysfunctions" ix

Andżelina Wolan-Nieroda, Jadwiga Dudziak, Mariusz Drużbicki, Bogumiła Pniak and Agnieszka Guzik
Effect of Dog-Assisted Therapy on Psychomotor Development of Children with Intellectual Disability
Reprinted from: *Children* **2021**, *8*, 13, doi:10.3390/children8010013 1

Bryan M. Gee, Kimberly Lloyd, Jesse Sutton and Tyler McOmber
Weighted Blankets and Sleep Quality in Children with Autism Spectrum Disorders: A Single-Subject Design
Reprinted from: *Children* **2021**, *8*, 10, doi:10.3390/children8010010 21

Majewska Joanna, Szczepanik Magdalena, Bazarnik-Mucha Katarzyna, Szymczyk Daniel and Lenart-Domka Ewa
The Utility of Gait Deviation Index (GDI) and Gait Variability Index (GVI) in Detecting Gait Changes in Spastic Hemiplegic Cerebral Palsy Children Using Ankle–Foot Orthoses (AFO)
Reprinted from: *Children* **2020**, *7*, 149, doi:10.3390/children7100149 35

Pong Sub Youn, Kyun Hee Cho and Shin Jun Park
Changes in Ankle Range of Motion, Gait Function and Standing Balance in Children with Bilateral Spastic Cerebral Palsy after Ankle Mobilization by Manual Therapy
Reprinted from: *Children* **2020**, *7*, 142, doi:10.3390/children7090142 45

Hye-Jin Cho and Byoung-Hee Lee
Effect of Functional Progressive Resistance Exercise on Lower Extremity Structure, Muscle Tone, Dynamic Balance and Functional Ability in Children with Spastic Cerebral Palsy
Reprinted from: *Children* **2020**, *7*, 85, doi:10.3390/children7080085 57

Young-a Jeong and Byoung-Hee Lee
Effect of Action Observation Training on Spasticity, Gross Motor Function, and Balance in Children with Diplegia Cerebral Palsy
Reprinted from: *Children* **2020**, *7*, 64, doi:10.3390/children7060064 71

Wei-Sheng Lin, Shan-Ju Lin and Ting-Rong Hsu
Cognitive Assessment and Rehabilitation for Pediatric-Onset Multiple Sclerosis: A Scoping Review
Reprinted from: *Children* **2020**, *7*, 183, doi:10.3390/children7100183 81

About the Editors

Agnieszka Guzik (DMSc.—higher doctoral degree, Professor of the University of Rzeszów): From 2008 to 2016, Dr. Guzik worked as an assistant at the Department of Rehabilitation at the Institute of Physiotherapy, Faculty of Medicine of the University of Rzeszów. From 2016 to 2019, she was employed as an assistant professor at the Department of Rehabilitation at the Institute of Physiotherapy, Faculty of Medicine, University of Rzeszów. In December 2019, she received a higher doctoral degree in medical sciences (DMSc) in the discipline of Health Sciences, following a habilitation procedure held at the Medical University of Silesia. In January 2020, she was nominated for a position of Professor at the University of Rzeszów. From 2019, she has been the head of the laboratory for physiotherapy of adult patients with neurological and neurosurgical conditions, as well as the Dean's proxy at the College of Medical Sciences. In her research, she has been involved in numerous projects focusing on the assessment of gait in patients with hemiparesis following damage to the central nervous system and additionally designed to investigate the use of biological feedback methods in neurological rehabilitation. At the same time, she acquired professional experience as a physiotherapist. From 2011, she was employed in the Ars Medica clinic in Krasne, where she worked with patients representing various age groups and dysfunctions and during 2013–2014 in the Early Intervention Centre (OWI) in Rzeszów. Her research interests include gait analysis, neurological gait disorders, and neurorehabilitation.

Lidia Perenc (DMSc.—higher doctoral degree, Professor of the University of Rzeszów): Dr. Perenc is a graduate of the Medical University in Poznań. After obtaining the professional title of physician, she became a specialist in paediatrics and medical rehabilitation. In 2004, she received a doctorate in medical sciences at the Medical University in Katowice on the basis of a dissertation entitled "Somatic development of children operated because of meningo-myelocele". In 2018, she obtained the degree of the habilitated doctor at the Collegium Medicum of the Jagiellonian University in Krakow. Since 1999, she has been employed at the University of Rzeszów. Currently, she is the director of the Institute of Health Sciences of this university. She is also employed at the Ward of Neurological Rehabilitation for Children and Youth, Regional Clinical Hospital No. 2, in Rzeszow.

Mariusz Drużbicki (DMSc.—higher doctoral degree in Health Sciences, Professor of the University of Rzeszów): Dr. Drużbicki holds the following science degrees: Master's Degree in Physical Education, Physical Education Faculty, Major in Teaching, from the Academy of Physical Education in Cracow (1989); Master's Degree in Physiotherapy, Physical Education Faculty, Major in Physiotherapy, from the Academy of Physical Education in Cracow (1991); PhD in Physical Education Science Physiotherapy, from the Academy of Physical Education in Cracow (2004). In 2018, he became an Associate Professor of the Academy of Physical Education in Cracow; in 2019, he became a Professor at the University of Rzeszów. Regarding his employment by scientific entities, since 2008, he has been the Manager of the Biomechanics Workshop, Department of Orthopedics and Traumatology, Medical Faculty, University of Rzeszów; since 2016, he has been the Manager of the Laboratory of Innovative Biofeedback Methods at the Centre for Innovative Research in Medical and Natural Sciences at the Medical Faculty, University of Rzeszów; since 2019, he has been the Manager and Chair of Physiotherapy at the Medical College of Rzeszów University; since 2001, he has been a Senior Assistant at the Rehabilitation Ward of County Hospital nr 2 in Rzeszów; since 2012, he has been the Manager of Physiotherapy at County Clinical Hospital nr 2 in Rzeszów. His main directions of research are neurorehabilitation, biomechanics, and gait analysis.

Preface to "Disorders of Motor, Somatic and Cognitive Development in Children with Neurodysfunctions"

Dysfunctions in a child's nervous system may be caused by numerous factors: genetic, physical, chemical, or environmental. The prevalence of neurodysfunctions in pediatric populations is relatively high compared to defects of other systems. This is linked to the fact that the development of the specific structures of the nervous system occurs over a relatively long period of time, during which the processes are affected by harmful factors. It may be difficult to accurately identify the cause, even in half of the children affected by the condition. The dysfunctions of the nervous system may have an impact on locomotion, somatic growth, and cognitive and social development. Therefore, children and adolescents with neurodysfunctions require continuous, comprehensive rehabilitation, covering not only motor functions but also mental and social ones. We hope that this book will reach a wide range of readers who have a professional interest in children and adolescents with neurodysfunctions. It will certainly be useful to physiotherapists, medical doctors, psychologists, and all members of interdisciplinary therapeutic teams.

Agnieszka Guzik, Lidia Perenc, Mariusz Drużbicki
Editors

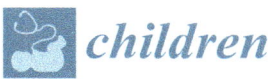

Article

Effect of Dog-Assisted Therapy on Psychomotor Development of Children with Intellectual Disability

Andżelina Wolan-Nieroda [1,*], Jadwiga Dudziak [1], Mariusz Drużbicki [1], Bogumiła Pniak [2] and Agnieszka Guzik [1]

1. Department of Physiotherapy, Institute of Health Sciences, College of Medical Sciences, University of Rzeszów, 35-959 Rzeszow, Poland; dudziaku3653@wp.pl (J.D.); mdruzb@ur.edu.pl (M.D.); agnieszkadepa2@wp.pl (A.G.)
2. Spa and Rehabilitation Hospital "EXCELSIOR", 38-440 Iwonicz Zdrój, Poland; gabipniak@vp.pl
* Correspondence: wolan.a@gmail.com

Received: 30 November 2020; Accepted: 25 December 2020; Published: 29 December 2020

Abstract: Background: Although dog-assisted therapy (DAT) has been used for years, there is still a scarcity of research findings confirming efficacy of the method. The current study was designed to assess effects of DAT on psychomotor development of children with mild intellectual disabilities. Material and method: The study involved 60 children with mild intellectual disabilities, aged 10–13 years, divided into a group participating in a 10-month DAT program, and the control group. Four tests were applied, i.e., finger identification, postural imitation, kinaesthesia, and Bourdon-Wiersma Dot Cancellation Test. The examinations were carried out before the start and at the end of the DAT, and at a two-month follow-up. Results: The results obtained by the DAT group in all the four tests, at all the three timepoints, were not the same ($p < 0.001$). No statistically significant differences were found in the measurement at the end of the therapy between the DAT group and the controls. On the other hand, the DAT group achieved significantly better scores ($p = 0.001$ and $p = 0.001$), compared to the control, in the follow-up measurements two months after the end of the therapy in postural imitation and finger identification tests. Conclusions: Some of the scores achieved by the children in the DAT group improved in the measurements performed over time. Two months after the therapy ended, the children in the DAT group presented greater gains in motor planning (postural imitation test) and in the sense of touch, attention, and concentration (finger identification test), compared to the control group. Although the measurement performed immediately after the therapy did not show significant differences between the DAT group and the controls, the examination carried out at the two-month follow-up identified long-term gains in the treatment group in the domain of motor planning (postural imitation test).

Keywords: dog-assisted therapy; intellectual disability; psychomotor disorders; child developmental; kinesthesis; cognition disorders; dogs

1. Introduction

Positive effects of Animal Assisted Therapy (AAT) on various physical and mental characteristics have been reported worldwide in the last 20 years. More specifically, many studies suggest that Dog Assisted Therapy (DAT) produces positive results in children with various developmental disorders, contributing to their ability to concentrate and to feel motivated for work [1–3]. Furthermore, research investigating effectiveness of AAT in relation to patients' social skills showed that interventions of this type favourably affected communication and social interactions between individuals with intellectual disability [3]. AAT is not only helpful as regards communication and basic activities of daily living. It has also been shown that in children with intellectual disability it may beneficially affect gross motor skills, since it can effectively boost a sense of motivation for exercise [4]. Dog-Assisted Therapy, also known as canine-assisted therapy or contact therapy, is gaining popularity and is well-tested as a form of complementary treatment [3–5]. Therapy dogs are used in rehabilitation of patients with motor and intellectual disabilities [5]. Contact therapy involving dogs is one of the methods that may be employed to promote the process of rehabilitation and recovery. Dogs are effectively used in treatment of individuals with disabilities or concentration and attention disorders because they favourably affect the psychophysical and socio-physical domains. Interaction with these animals reduces anxiety, simulates sense organs, increases vocabulary resources, and improves contact with the environment [6,7]. DAT enables children to improve gross motor skills, own-body perception as well as fine motor skills. It favourably affects cognitive skills, such as concentration, perceptivity, ability to take decisions, as well as ability to adequately perceive and respond to a given situation. Games and fun activities taking place during DAT facilitate learning and consolidation of such notions as colours, sizes, numbers, differences, and similarities. A review of the related literature shows that DAT also contributes to better psychomotor efficiency [8–10]. Studies by Jorge et al. showed positive effects of DAT in children's motor development, particularly balance, motor planning, and spatial orientation [11]. It appears that DAT is particularly successful as a way to help individuals with intellectual disabilities and improve their psychomotor efficiency. Interaction with an animal leads to enhancement of neurotransmission in the human, which initiates decrease in blood pressure and induces relaxation. This association may be beneficial in reducing arousal as well as psychological symptoms of chronic diseases, including physical and mental disabilities [12,13]. A study by Scorzato et al., assessing effects of DAT in individuals with intellectual disability, showed significant improvement related to a number of cognitive factors, including focus on movement, visuomotor coordination, exploratory games, and imitation of motion. The effects of the therapy did not depend on the subjects' age and degree of intellectual disability [14]. Gocheva et al. also reported statistically significant findings related to attention and concentration in patients with brain injury participating in DAT [15]. Kongable et al. observed positive effects of DAT in tactile and visual perception as well as verbalisation [13]. Systematic participation in appropriately structured activities involving a dog makes it possible for children using this type of therapy to improve their physical and mental condition. DAT promotes overall physical activity and motor capacities. Children with intellectual disability participating in exercise frequently have problems with motor activity, they are sluggish and unwilling to move. A dog motivates them to take action; they approach the animal to say hello, and they focus their attention on the dog. DAT improves precision of movements, as a result of which the child gains greater motor control [16]. This is also an excellent form of rehabilitation for a child. Presence of a dog helps in performance of self-care activities and reduces emotional tension. "Depending on the child's needs, during dog-assisted therapy session the child may perform a number of exercises focusing on gross motor skills, manual efficiency and visual perception" [17]. Contact therapy involving a dog facilitates own-body schema orientation, allowing the child to understand the structure of both animal and human body, and to improve their motor efficiency, as a result of exercise performed together with the dog and through stimulation of the senses of vision, hearing, and touch as well as practice of attention and concentration. Numerous studies demonstrated effectiveness and usefulness of animals in therapy [12–19]. An animal does not only help to calm down and to develop one's social behaviours but also constitutes a source of motivation [20]. Owing to their inherent qualities, animals may induce child's interest and may stimulate a variety of sensory functions through sounds, movement, smell, and touch. Their activity is simple, repeatable, and non-verbal; as a result, it is more accessible even to individuals with language dysfunctions [21]. Animals are a source of and the purpose for attention [22]. Efforts to systematically categorise the ways humans are affected by animals made it possible to distinguish a few mechanisms:

- Affective—related to feelings aroused in a person by the animal;
- Psychological stimulation—interaction with the animal, stimulating social behaviours and cognitive functions;
- Recreational—related to activation of motor functions and motor planning [23,24].

Therapy intended for a child with intellectual disability should be intensive and multidimensional; it should boost the development of and strengthen the child's intellectual functioning, as a result potentially increasing his/her independence. Because of this, therapy should be designed to stimulate perception-related functions of the brain, concentration, and attention, to improve motor functions, to promote development of speech and communication skills [20]. The methods facilitating rehabilitation of children with intellectual disability include DAG, which is intended to stimulate development in all the domains and promote improvement in motor capacities. The above review of literature suggests that DAT favourably affects concentration and attention [9], motor planning [15], spatial orientation [15] as well as sense of touch [21]. DAT is a widely used form of supplementary treatment. However, few reports so far have specifically focused on the effects of this type of intervention in children with intellectual disability [24,25]. Therefore, the present study aimed to investigate whether or not long-term/delayed effects of DAT would impact children's performance during a period when they did not participate in education and rehabilitation programs.

In view of the above, the study was designed to assess psychomotor efficiency, reflected by the factors of attention and concentration, motor planning, spatial orientation, and sense of touch in children with mild intellectual disability participating in DAT and in controls receiving no such therapy, immediately after the period of education and rehabilitation and following a period during which the children did not receive DAT and did not participate in education and rehabilitation.

Hypotheses:

Hypothesis 1. *Children with intellectual disability, participating in an educational program supplemented with DAT, achieve improvement in attention and concentration, motor planning, spatial orientation, and sense of touch, in assessments carried out at the end of the educational program and at a two-month follow up.*

Hypothesis 2. *Improvement in the DAT study group is significantly greater than in the non-DAT control group.*

Hypothesis 3. *Effects of education supplemented with DAT are long-lasting. Children additionally receiving DAT after a two-month break in the education program present greater improvement compared to the non-DAT control group.*

2. Materials and Methods

2.1. Participants

The study was conducted in a special educational facility in the Podkarpackie Region, Poland, and involved 60 children with mild intellectual disability, mean age 11 years ± 2.3 years. Eligibility criteria included: Mild intellectual disability (intelligence quotient of 50–70 according to Wechsler Intelligence Scale) [26,27], special school education, age 10–13 years, and parent's/legal guardian's consent to participate. The study protocol excluded children with moderate to severe intellectual disability with cognitive deficits impairing the ability to understand and follow instructions. Other exclusion criteria were defined as follows: Co-existing autism, cerebral palsy, total visual and hearing impairment, muscular dystrophy and neurological disorders such as brain injury and epilepsy. Prospective subjects were disqualified from the study if their parents/legal guardians failed to grant consent for participation.

2.2. Flow of the Subjects through the Study

One hundred children were examined successively, as they were admitted to a special educational facility in the Podkarpackie Region, Poland. Ultimately 60 children were enrolled for the study. Out of the 40 children who were not qualified for the programme, 28 failed to meet the inclusion criteria, and 12 refused to participate. All the subjects completed the final examination. Figure 1 shows the flow of the subjects through the study.

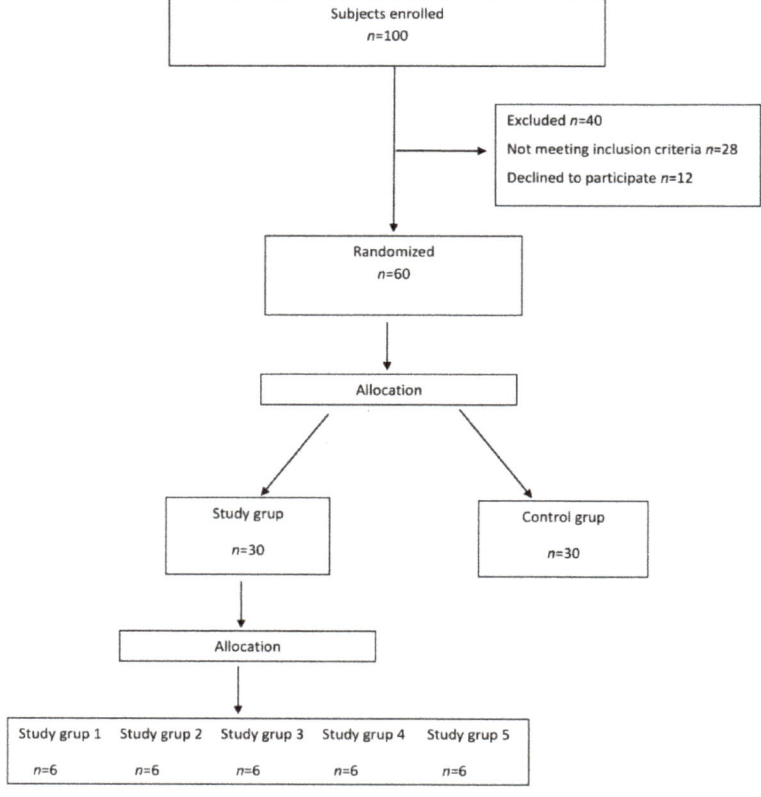

Figure 1. Flow of subjects through the study.

2.3. Study Design

Single blind trial design was applied with randomised assignment of participants to one of the two parallel groups comprising a total of 60 children with intellectual disability, attending the same special educational facility in the Podkarpackie Region, Poland. Simple randomization was used, i.e., randomisation based on a single sequence of random assignments. The most common and basic method of simple randomisation was applied, which involved flipping a coin [28], the side of the coin (i.e., heads—DTA group, tails—control group) determined the assignment of each subject. First degree randomisation, i.e., random selection of subjects to two groups, the DTA group and the control group, whereby the children were allocated either to the group receiving DTA (the DTA group—30 children, 19 girls and 11 boys) or to the group that did not participate in the DAT program (the control group—30 children, 20 girls and 10 boys). Subsequently the DAT group was randomly divided by second degree randomisation, i.e., the subjects were assigned to five therapeutic subgroups, each comprising 6 children, relative to the procedures applied in the DAT. The subgroups had common characteristics in terms of functionality level (all the children presented the same functionality level in activities of daily living expressed by Barthel Index of 80–85 points), and cognitive level (mild intellectual disability—intelligence quotient of 50–70 according to Wechsler Intelligence Scale). All the children met all the inclusion criteria. The DAT program was continued for 10 months, with 45-min sessions taking place once a week.

2.4. Study Protocol

The protocol of this randomised study was approved by the local Bioethics Commission of the Medical Faculty (4 February 2017). The data presented in this article were obtained in a two-armed randomised controlled trial. Informed consent for the children's participation in the study was obtained in writing from their parents or legal guardians. Experimental conditions were in compliance with the Declaration of Helsinki. No adverse events were observed during the study. Inclusion/exclusion criteria were met. No intentional deviations from the protocol were observed during the study.

2.5. Measurements

The assessments were carried out three times: At the start of the DAT program (Exam 1), at the end of the therapy program (i.e., after 10 months) (Exam 2), and at a two-month follow-up (Exam 3). The following research tools were used:

- Bourdon–Wiersma Dot Cancellation Test—assessing concentration and attention. The subject is shown a sheet with a sequence of various letters and digits and is asked to quickly cross out specific letters, e.g., e and r, within 3 min. The result is based on the total number of characters crossed out correctly, and a total number of characters skipped and selected mistakenly. Each type of error may be indicative of an impairment in different processes of attention, e.g., weakening. A maximum of 102 points can be scored. In the entire sheet, the digit 6 appears 102 times. One point is scored for each digit 6 crossed out correctly [29].
- The Southern California Sensory Integration Tests (SCSIT Battery) proposed by J. Ayres, based on Southern California Sensory Integration Tests Manual, Los Angeles, Calif., Western Psychological Services [30,31]. The battery is designed to evaluate sensory integration by assessing e.g., kinaesthetic sense, perception of tactile stimuli, ability to visualise tactile sensations without visual control, ability to sense the location of tactile stimuli, as well as movement planning. The subtests used in the present study include postural imitation test—assessing motor planning and sequencing. A maximum of 12 points can be scored. The child is awarded 1 point if they correctly assume a position or 0 points if they fail to assume the position; finger identification test—assessing the sense of touch, attention and concentration. A maximum of 16 points can be scored, one point for each correct answer; as well as kinaesthesia test—assessing kinaesthetic sense, spatial positioning of extremities, and memory. A maximum of 24 points can be scored. The child is to indicate 12 locations where tactile stimuli were applied. Two points are scored for each correctly indicated location. If the child points to the correct part of the limb but not to the precise location, they score 1 point. If they fail to correctly indicate the location or the part of the limb, they score 0 points.

2.6. Procedure

The DAT program was continued for 10 months, with 45-min sessions held once a week. The sessions were carried out in groups of six children and aimed to improve functioning of memory and attention processes, to ensure adequate level of motivation, to increase sense of security and self-confidence in the presence of the dog, to boost the ability to cope with difficult emotions, to improve motor function and the sense of balance, and to reduce the sense of anxiety and loneliness through contact with the therapist and the dog. Some of the originally planned sessions had to be cancelled due to the patient's or the therapist's illness. All the DAT sessions were conducted in a therapy room in the premises of the facility. No therapy session had to be stopped earlier and no undesired events occurred. Needs of each patient and the goals of DAT (Table 1) were taken into account. The sessions in each of the five groups followed the same DAT program. In addition to that the children in the DAT group as well as the controls participated in a conventional treatment program, which included rehabilitation (individual practice focusing on endurance, correction, balance as well as strengthening of postural and respiratory muscles), speech therapy, as well as educational, artistic, and musical activities.

Table 1. Description of Dog-Assisted Therapy (DAT) sessions.

Month/Group 1–5	Week	Introductory Activities, Making Contact with the Dog, Grooming and Taking Care of the Dog	Practice of Gross Motor Skills, Balance and Motor Coordination	Practice of Fine Motor Skills	Exercises Involving Memory, Attention and Concentration	Exercises Stimulating Haptic Perception. Normalisation of Muscle Tone	Improvement of Body Schema and Spatial Orientation	Duration of DAT per Week
I	I	10	10	15		10		45
	II	10	10		15		10	45
	III	10	10	15		10		45
	IV	10	10		15		10	45
	Total	40 min	40 min	30 min	30 min	20 min	20 min	
II	I	5	10	15		10	5	45
	II	5	10		15	10	5	45
	III	5	10	15		10	5	45
	IV	5	10		15	10	5	45
	Total	20 min	40 min	30 min	30 min	40 min	20 min	
III	I	5	10		15	10	5	45
	II	5	10	15		10	5	45
	III	5	10		15	10	5	45
	IV	5	10	15		10	5	45
	Total	20 min	40 min	30 min	30 min	40 min	20 min	
IV	I	5	10	15		10	5	45
	II	5	10		15	10	5	45
	III	5	10	15		10	5	45
	IV	5	10		15	10	5	45
	Total	20 min	40 min	30 min	30	40 min	20 min	
V	I	5	10	15		10	5	45
	II	5	10		15	10	5	45
	III	5	10	15		10	5	45
	IV	5	10		15	10	5	45
	Total	20 min	40 min	30 min	30	40 min	20 min	
VI	I	5	10	15		10	5	45
	II	5	10		15	10	5	45
	III	5	10	15		10	5	45
	IV	5	10		15	10	5	45
	Total	20 min	40 min	30 min	30	40 min	20 min	
VII	I	5	10	15		10	5	45
	II	5	10		15	10	5	45
	III	5	10	15		10	5	45
	IV	5	10		15	10	5	45
	Total	20 min	40 min	30 min	30	40 min	20 min	
VIII	I	5	10	15		10	5	45
	II	5	10		15	10	5	45
	III	5	10	15		10	5	45
	IV	5	10		15	10	5	45
	Total	20 min	40 min	30 min	30 min	40 min	20 min	
IX	I	5	10	15		10	5	45
	II	5	10		15	10	5	45
	III	5	10	15		10	5	45
	IV	5	10		15	10	5	45
	Total	20 min	40 min	30 min	30 min	40 min	20 min	
X	I	5	10	15		10	5	45
	II	5	10		15	10	5	45
	III	5	10	15		10	5	45
	IV	5	10		15	10	5	45
	Total	20 min	40 min	30 min	30 min	40 min	20 min	
Total duration of DAT		3 h 40 min	6 h 40 min	5 h	5 h	6 h 20 min	3 h 20 min	

In our study, the DAT program was supervised by a team of experienced therapists for years providing services to children with intellectual disability.

2.7. Statistical Analysis

Statistical analyses were performed using Statistica 13.1. software developed by StatSoft Polska. The obtained results of the examinations did not meet the criteria for parametric tests, i.e., normality of distribution of the relevant variables, due to which alternative non-parametric tests were applied in the analyses. Compatibility of the distributions with normal distribution was verified using Shapiro–Wilk test. Comparison of the results achieved by the children in the DAT group in the consecutive timepoints relative to the therapy (measurement over time) was performed using Friedman's ANOVA, Dunn's test being a suitable post-hoc analytic tool. Comparison of the results within the two groups (DAT and control) was performed using Mann-Whitney U-test. Differences in the therapeutic effects (short- and long-term) in the same group of subjects were examined using paired samples Wilcoxon test. Statistical significance was assumed if $p < 0.05$.

2.8. Sample Size

The minimum size of the sample was calculated taking into account the number of children with intellectual disability attending the special educational facility in the Podkarpackie Region, Poland, annually. A fraction size of 0.9 was used, with a maximum error of 5% [32–35], a sample size of 58 children was obtained. The study involved 60 children. The following formula was applied to determine the minimum sample size:

$$N_{min} = \frac{N p (\alpha^2 \cdot f(1-f))}{N p \cdot e^2 + \alpha^2 \cdot f(1-f)}$$

N_{min}—minimum sample size
N_P—size of the population sampled
α—confidence level for the results, value of Z-score in normal distribution for the assumed significance level, e.g., 1.96
f—fraction size
e—assumed maximum error expressed with a fractional number, e.g., 3% is expressed as 0.03

3. Results

Based on the examinations, statistical differences between the scores observed at the three timepoints—at the start of the DAT (Exam 1), at the end of the therapy program (i.e., after 10 months) (Exam 2), and at a two-month follow-up (Exam 3)—were assessed in the relevant group of children.

Hypothesis 1. *Children with intellectual disability, participating in an educational program supplemented with DAT, achieve improvement in attention and concentration, motor planning, spatial orientation, and sense of touch, in assessments carried out at the end of the educational program and at a two-month follow up.*

It was shown that the results obtained by the DAT group in the category of finger identification, measured at the three timepoints (before the DAT, at the end of the DAT, and at a two-month follow-up) were not the same ($p < 0.001$). In order to identify statistically significant differences between the measurements at the specific timepoints, a post-hoc analysis was performed using Dunn's test, appropriate for Friedman's ANOVA. The analysis showed differences in the results between the measurements performed before and immediately after the therapy, measurements before the DAT and at the two-month follow-up, as well as measurements immediately after the DAT and at the two-month follow-up. Each subsequent measurement showed higher scores. Before the therapy the children achieved the lowest results; in the measurement immediately after the therapy there was a statistically significant increase and subsequently, at the two-month follow-up, again the scores were significantly higher relative to the short-term effect (Table 2).

Table 2. Identification—analyses of the measurements performed over time.

Finger Identification	Basic Descriptive Statistics										
	Number	Mean	−95% CI	+95% CI	Median	Min.	Max.	First Quartile	Third Quartile	StDev	Effect Size
Before DAT-I	30	8.57	7.35	9.79	8.00	4.00	13.00	6.00	12.00	3.27	
Difference II-I	30	1.20	0.50	1.90	1.50	−6.00	4.00	0.00	2.00	1.86	0.47
Immediately after DAT-II	30	9.77	8.62	10.91	9.50	4.00	13.00	7.00	13.00	3.06	
Difference III-II	30	1.97	1.16	2.78	1.00	0.00	7.00	0.00	4.00	2.17	0.84
Two-month follow-up-III	30	11.73	11.13	12.34	12.00	8.00	13.00	11,.00	13.00	1.62	
Difference III-I	30	3.17	2.27	4.07	3.00	0.00	8.00	1.00	5.00	2.41	1.29
p	Chi^2 Friedman's ANOVA (N = 30, df = 2) = 41.02326 $p < 0.001$ Absolute differences between rank sums are (approximately) significant if > 18.5436877917081 at a significance level = 0.05										
	Before DAT			Immediately after DAT			Two-month follow-up				
Before DAT	—			21			42				
Immediately after DAT	21			—			21				
Two-month follow-up	42			21			—				

CI: confidence interval.

It was shown that the results obtained by the DAT group in the category of postural imitation, measured at the three timepoints (before the DAT, at the end of the DAT, and at a two-month follow-up) were not the same ($p < 0.001$). The post hoc (Dunn's) test showed there were differences between the results measured before DAT and at the two-month follow-up, as well as the results measured immediately after the DAT and at the two-month follow-up. The analysis did not confirm statistically significant differences between the results measured before the DAT and immediately after the DAT. The measurement before the DAT identified the lowest scores. Immediately after the DAT, the scores improved only slightly, however the further increase in the results, reflected by the difference in the measurements immediately after the DAT and at the two-month follow-up, was statistically significant. The result identified in the final measurement differed significantly from the baseline (Table 3).

Table 3. Postural imitation—analyses of the measurements performed over time.

Postural Imitation	Basic Descriptive Statistics										
	Number	Mean	−95% CI	+95% CI	Median	Min.	Max.	First Quartile	Third Quartile	StDev	Effect Size
Before DAT-I	30	7.57	6.32	8.81	8.50	3.00	11.00	4.00	11.00	3.34	
Difference II-I	30	0.83	0.51	1.16	1.00	0.00	3.00	0.00	1.00	0.87	0.26
Immediately after DAT-II	30	8.40	7.26	9.54	10.50	3.00	12.00	5.00	11.00	3.05	
Difference III-II	30	3.03	1.88	4.19	1.50	−3.00	11.00	1.00	5.00	3.09	1.29
Two-month follow-up-III	30	11.43	10.82	12.04	12.00	6.00	15.00	12.00	12.00	1.63	
Difference III-I	30	3.87	2.58	5.15	3.00	−3.00	12.00	1.00	6.00	3.44	1.55
p	Chi^2 Friedman's ANOVA (N = 30, df = 2) = 46.85437 $p < 0.001$ Absolute differences between rank sums are (approximately) significant if > 18.5436877917081 at a significance level = 0.05										
	Before DAT			Immediately after DAT			Two-month follow-up				
Before DAT	—			17.5			48.5				
Immediately after DAT	17.5			—			31				
Two-month follow-up	48.5			31			—				

It was shown that the results obtained by the DAT group in the category of kinaesthesia, measured at the three timepoints (before the DAT, at the end of the DAT, and at a two-month follow-up) were not the same ($p < 0.001$). The post hoc (Dunn's) test showed there were differences between the results measured before DAT and immediately after the DAT, as well as the results measured before the DAT and at the two-month follow-up. The analysis did not confirm statistically significant differences between the results measured immediately after the DAT and at the two-month follow-up. The measurement before the DAT identified the lowest scores. Subsequently, there was a significant increase in the measurement immediately after the DAT and the effect was maintained, despite a small decrease, in the measurement at the two-month follow-up (Table 4).

Table 4. Kinaesthesia—analyses of the measurements performed over time.

Kinaesthesia	Basic Descriptive Statistics										
	Number	Mean	−95% CI	+95% CI	Median	Min.	Max.	First Quartile	Third Quartile	StDev	Effect Size
Before DAT-I	30	15.07	12.54	17.60	17.00	1.00	24.00	8.00	20.00	6.77	
Difference II-I	30	1.70	1.07	2.33	1.00	0.00	6.00	0.00	3.00	1.68	0.25
Immediately after DAT-II	30	16.77	14.19	19.34	19.00	2.00	24.00	11.00	24.00	6.90	
Difference III-II	30	−0.50	−2.07	1.07	0.00	−12.00	8.00	−3.00	2.00	4.22	0.08
Two-month follow-up-III	30	16.27	14.09	18.44	17.50	4.00	24.00	12.00	21.00	5.82	
Difference III-I	30	1.20	−0.48	2.88	2.00	−12.00	9.00	0.00	4.00	4.51	0.19
p	Chi^2 Friedman's ANOVA (N = 30, df = 2) = 19.38947 $p < 0.001$ Absolute differences between rank sums are (approximately) significant if > 18.5436877917081 at a significance level = 0.05										
	Before DAT			Immediately after DAT			Two-month follow-up				
Before DAT	—			27			25.5				
Immediately after DAT	27			—			1.5				
Two-month follow-up	25.5			1.5			—				

It was shown that the results obtained by the DAT group in the Bourdon–Wiersma Dot Cancellation Test, measured at the three timepoints (before the DAT, at the end of the DAT, and at a two-month follow-up) were not the same ($p < 0.001$). The post hoc (Dunn's) test showed there were differences between the results measured before DAT and immediately after the DAT, as well as the results measured before the DAT and at the two-month follow-up. The analysis did not confirm statistically significant differences between the results measured immediately after the DAT and at the two-month follow-up. The measurement before the DAT identified the lowest scores. Subsequently there was a significant increase in the measurement immediately after the DAT and the effect was maintained, but without a significant increase, in the measurement at the two-month follow-up (Table 5).

Table 5. Bourdon–Wiersma Dot Cancellation—analyses of the measurements performed over time.

Bourdon-Wiersma Dot Cancellation Test	Basic Descriptive Statistics										
	Number	Mean	−95% CI	+95% CI	Median	Min.	Max.	First Quartile	Third Quartile	StDev	Effect Size
Before DAT-I	30	25.70	18.41	32.99	19.50	2.00	54.00	8.00	52.00	19.52	
Difference II-I	30	3.30	2.21	4.39	3.50	−1.00	10.00	1.00	5.00	2.91	0.16
Immediately after DAT-II	30	29.00	21.20	36.80	24.00	2.00	60.00	9.00	54.00	20.90	
Difference III-II	30	4.50	−1.59	10.59	5.50	−54.00	45.00	0.00	8.00	16.32	0.21
Two-month follow-up-III	30	33.50	25.56	41.44	33.00	5.00	60.00	10.00	59.00	21.26	
Difference III-I	30	7.80	1.85	13.75	8.00	−47.00	50.00	2.00	12.00	15.94	0.38
p	Chi^2 Friedman's ANOVA (N = 30, df = 2) = 29.05556 $p < 0.001$ Absolute differences between rank sums are (approximately) significant if > 18.5436877917081 at a significance level = 0.05										
	Before DAT			Immediately after DAT			Two-month follow-up				
Before DAT	—			25.5			39				
Immediately after DAT	25.5			—			13.5				
Two-month follow-up	39			13.5			—				

Hypothesis 2. *Improvement in the DAT study group is significantly greater than in the non-DAT control group.*

The next part of the analyses involved comparison of the results achieved by the children in the DAT group at each stage of the therapy program to the scores of the children in the control group.

As regards finger identification the DAT group and the controls did not differ in the measurement before and immediately after the DAT, however the measurement two months after the DAT was completed showed statistically significant differences between the groups ($p < 0.001$), reflecting greater gains in the DAT group. The finding was confirmed by assessing effect size with Cohen's d. Hence, the short-term changes in the two groups were comparable, however the performance of the DAT group reflected statistically better long-term effects possibly resulting from the therapy (Table 6).

No differences related to kinaesthesia were found between the DAT group and the controls in the measurements before and immediately after the DAT, and at the two-month follow-up. The finding was confirmed by assessing effect size with Cohen's d (Table 7).

The scores in postural imitation test showed the DAT group and the controls did not differ in the measurements before and immediately after the DAT. On the other hand, the measurement at a two-month follow-up identified statistically significant differences ($p < 0.001$), with higher scores achieved by the DAT group. The finding was confirmed by assessing effect size with Cohen's d. Hence, the short-term improvement in the two groups was comparable, however the scores of the DAT group seem to reflect statistically higher long-term effects of the therapy (Table 8).

As regards the Bourdon–Wiersma Dot Cancellation Test, the DAT group and the controls did not differ in the measurements at any stage of the therapy program. The finding was confirmed by assessing effect size with Cohen's d (Table 9).

Hypothesis 3. *Effects of education supplemented with DAT are long-lasting. Children additionally receiving DAT after a two-month break in the education program present greater improvement compared to the non-DAT control group.*

Comparative analysis examined relationships between measurement II and I (short-term effect—before the DAT versus immediately after the DAT) and measurement III and II (long-term effect—immediately after the DAT versus two-month follow-up).

As for the effect size identified in measurements I and II, as well as II and III, no significant differences were found in finger identification and in the Bourdon–Wiersma Dot Cancellation Test ($p > 0.05$). This means that immediately after DAT and at the two-month follow-up the children achieved similar results.

Assessment of the scores in postural imitation test showed that the long-term effect, reflected by measurement III versus II, was significantly greater than the short-term effect.

The related analyses of the scores in the kinaesthesia test showed a positive short-term effect and a negative long-term effect ($p = 0.009$), (Table 10). However, the previous findings (Table 3) showed that this decrease was not significant from the viewpoint of the therapy effectiveness because the final effect was similar to that observed immediately after the DAT and the scores were higher than those achieved before the DAT (Table 10).

Table 6. Finger identification—comparison of the scores achieved by the DAT group and the controls.

Finger Identification	Number	Mean	−95% CI	+95% CI	Median	Min.	Max.	First Quartile	Third Quartile	StDev	Cohen's d	Mann-Whitney U-Test-Z	p	Effect Size
DAT group—before therapy	30	8.57	7.35	9.79	8.00	4.00	13.00	6.00	12.00	3.27	0.02	0.04	0.971	0.02
Control group	30	8.50	7.53	9.47	8.00	4.00	13.00	6.00	11.00	2.60				
Immediately after DAT	30	9.40	8.49	10.31	10.00	4.00	14.00	8.00	11.00	2.43	0.04	0.57	0.564	0.04
Control group	30	9.50	8.49	10.51	9.50	5.00	15.00	8.00	12.00	2.70				
Two-month follow-up	30	11.73	11.13	12.34	12.00	8.00	13.00	11.00	13.00	1.62	1.15	3.89	<0.001	1.15
Control group	30	9.40	8.49	10.31	10.00	4.00	14.00	8.00	11.00	2.43				

Table 7. Kinaesthesia—comparison of DAT group scores achieved over time to the results of the controls.

Kinaesthesia	Number	Mean	−95% CI	+95% CI	Median	Min.	Max.	First Quartile	Third Quartile	StDev	Cohen's d	Mann-Whitney U-Test-Z	p	Effect Size
DAT group—before therapy	30	15.07	12.54	17.60	17.00	1.00	24.00	8.00	20.00	6.77	0.30	1.18	0.240	0.30
Control group	30	13.23	12.00	6.00	24.00	8.00	17.00	5.35	17.00	5.35				
Immediately after DAT	30	16.77	14.19	19.34	19.00	2.00	24.00	11.00	24.00	6.90	0.40	1.63	0.104	0.40
Control group	30	14.30	12.25	16.35	14.00	6.00	25.00	10.00	18.00	5.48				
Two-month follow-up	30	16.27	14.09	18.44	17.50	4.00	24.00	12.00	21.00	5.82	0.41	1.60	0.110	0.41
Control group	30	14.00	12.04	15.96	13.50	5.00	25.00	10.00	17.00	5.26				

Table 8. Postural imitation—comparison of DAT group scores achieved over time to the results of the controls.

Postural Imitation	Number	Mean	−95% CI	+95% CI	Median	Min.	Max.	First Quartile	Third Quartile	StDev	Cohen's d	Mann-Whitney U-Test-Z	p	Effect Size
DAT group—before therapy	30	7.57	6.32	8.81	8.50	3.00	11.00	4.00	11.00	3.34	0.35	−0.58	0.559	0.35
Control group	30	8.47	7.77	9.17	8.00	4.00	12.00	7.00	10.00	1.87				
Immediately after DAT	30	8.40	7.26	9.54	10.50	3.00	12.00	5.00	11.00	3.05	0.51	−0.86	0.387	0.51
Control group	30	9.80	8.88	10.72	10.00	5.00	15.00	9.00	11.00	2.46				
Two-month follow-up	30	11.43	10.82	12.04	12.00	6.00	15.00	12.00	12.00	1.63	0.94	3.78	<0.001	0.94
Control group	30	9.37	8.34	10.39	9.00	4.00	15.00	8.00	11.00	2.75				

Table 9. Bourdon–Wiersma Dot Cancellation Test—comparison of DAT group scores achieved over time to the results of the controls.

Bourdon-Wiersma Dot Cancellation Test	Number	Mean	−95% CI	+95% CI	Median	Min.	Max.	First Quartile	Third Quartile	StDev	Cohen's d	Mann-Whitney U-Test–Z	p	Effect Size
DAT group—before therapy	30	25.70	18.41	32.99	19.50	2.00	54.00	8.00	52.00	19.52	0.12	−1.03	0.301	0.12
Control group	30	27.67	23.01	32.32	23.50	6.00	54.00	19.00	36.00	12.47				
Immediately after DAT	30	29.00	21.20	36.80	24.00	2.00	60.00	9.00	54.00	20.90	0.00	−0.40	0.690	0.00
Control group	30	28.93	24.33	33.53	26.00	7.00	54.00	20.00	37.00	12.32				
Two-month follow-up	30	33.50	25.56	41.44	33.00	5.00	60.00	10.00	59.00	21.26	0.31	0.79	0.429	0.31
Control group	30	28.17	23.42	32.91	26.00	7.00	54.00	19.00	36.00	12.71				

Table 10. Comparison of the therapy effects, short-term and long-term.

		Number	Mean	−95% CI	+95% CI	Median	Min.	Max.	First Quartile	Third Quartile	StDev	Cohen's d	Paired Samples Wilcoxon Test–Z	p	Effect Size
Finger identification	Difference II-I	30	1.20	0.50	1.90	1.50	−6.00	4.00	0.00	2.00	1.86	−0.38	0.99	0.322	0.38
	Difference III-II	30	1.97	1.16	2.78	1.00	0.00	7.00	0.00	4.00	2.17				
Kinaesthesia	Difference II-I	30	1.70	1.07	2.33	1.00	0.00	6.00	0.00	3.00	1.68	0.75	2.60	0.009	0.75
	Difference III-II	30	−0.50	−2.07	1.07	0.00	−12.00	8.00	−3.00	2.00	4.22				
Postural imitation	Difference II-I	30	0.83	0.51	1.16	1.00	0.00	3.00	0.00	1.00	0.87	1.11	3.41	0.001	1.11
	Difference III-II	30	3.03	1.88	4.19	1.50	−3.00	11.00	1.00	5.00	3.09				
Bourdon-Wierman Test	Difference II-I	30	3.30	2.21	4.39	3.50	−1.00	10.00	1.00	5.00	2.91	0.12	0.84	0.400	0.12
	Difference III-II	30	4.50	−1.59	10.59	5.50	−54.00	45.00	0.00	8.00	16.32				

4. Discussion

The present study investigated effects of DAT on psychomotor development of children with mild intellectual disability. Even though DAT has been used for years, the related gains from this type of intervention have rarely been assessed in children with intellectual disability [8,14]. Conversely, a quick review of the literature shows a number of publications assessing effects of DAT on the development of children with cerebral palsy, various motor disabilities, and autism [36–38].

The current study involved a group of children with mild intellectual disability, aged 10–13 years (mean age 11 years ± 2.3 years). The children presented poorer abilities reflected by scores in finger identification, postural imitation, and kinaesthesia tests, compared to healthy children in the same age group [30]. Bülent et al. assessed sensory integration and activities of daily living in children with developmental coordination disorder; the scores achieved by the study group in postural imitation tests were considerably lower, compared to the scores of their healthy peers. Similar results were obtained in localisation of tactile stimuli and kinaesthesia tests [39]. Schoemaker et al. reported similar findings in a study assessing perceptual skills in children with impaired coordination. Children from the study group achieved poorer scores in a test assessing tactile perception and attention [40].

The present study suggests that DAT contributes to improvement in concentration reflected by the scores in finger identification test and Bourdon–Wiersma Dot Cancellation test. Before the therapy, the children achieved the lowest results; in the measurement immediately after the therapy, there was a statistically significant increase. Likewise, François et al. in their publication discussed effects of DAT on the functioning of children with pervasive developmental disorders and reported that during the therapy the children focused mainly on the dog. When they were assisted by a therapy dog, they were able to concentrate better and they exhibited greater awareness of their social environment [39]. Reed et al. conducted a study focusing on DAT and its effectiveness in children with autism. Children with autism disorder participating in DAT were found with better ability to concentrate and focus their attention, had higher intellectual potential and ability to learn as well as decreased level of anxiety [41].

In accordance with the protocol of the current study, the DAT sessions were carried out in groups of six children, and aimed to improve functioning of memory and attention processes, to ensure adequate level of motivation, increase sense of security and self-confidence in the presence of the dog, boost the ability to cope with difficult emotions, improve motor function and the sense of balance, and reduce the sense of anxiety and loneliness through the contact with the therapist and the dog. The results achieved by the children in the DAT group in kinaesthetic sense, perception of tactile stimuli, ability to visualise tactile sensations without visual control, and ability to sense the location of tactile stimuli were significantly improved immediately after therapy. Nawrocka-Rohnka conducted a study involving children with cerebral palsy, autism, and intellectual disability. The DAT sessions were held in groups of three children. The greatest progress was observed in the ability to communicate commands (mean improvement by 37.89%). This result may reflect improved functioning related to both the intellectual domain—remembering the instruction and the sequence of gestures necessary in communicating commands—and the mental domain—development of the sense of self-efficacy and improved self-esteem. Another area of significant progress observed in that study was related to "expression on emotions" (mean improvement by 30.96%), corresponding to the socioemotional domain. The poorest effects were found in the area of "mobility" (mean improvement by 30.96%), corresponding to the motor domain [42].

In another study, Gee et al. investigated effects of DAT on motor efficiency of pre-schoolers with language disorders. The researchers assessed locomotion, balance, and coordination before and after DAT. The children achieved better scores when they were working in the presence of a dog [43]. In the current study, DAT sessions were designed to include practice of gross motor skills, balance, and motor coordination. The analysis did not confirm statistically significant differences between the results in motor planning measured before the DAT and immediately after the DAT. Importantly, however, the further improvement, reflected by the difference in the measurements immediately after the DAT and at the two-month follow-up, was statistically significant. The result identified in the final measurement at the two-month follow-up, differed significantly from the baseline. It is likely that this result is associated with the fact that the effects of DAT in the study group were strengthened by the children's involvement in basic and complex activities of daily living in home setting during summer holidays. The learning process in fact may have required more time, and the summer break, which involved a change of the environment, enabled a consolidation of the skills acquired during the 10 months, since they had to be "brought home" from the setting of the day care centre. Other researchers also observed that assistance of a dog during therapy sessions is associated with patients' greater motivation and confidence during therapeutic activities as well as improved motor skills following the therapy; the children are more independent and function more effectively in the daily life [44,45].

The current study compared effects of the therapy (short-term—at the end of a 10-month DAT and long-term—at the two-month follow-up). As for the effect size reflected by the relation between measurements I and II, as well as II and III, the long-term effect (measurement III versus II) was significantly greater than the short-term effect in the category of postural imitation while a reverse situation was observed in the results of kinaesthesia test. It can be assumed that the change identified at the end of the therapy program is directly associated with the effectiveness of DAT, while the significant change identified two months later may reflect the fact that during the therapy the children received a certain stimulus and learned new psychomotor skills, which required sufficient time to be further improved. Similar long-term effects of DAT were reported by Piek et al. who concluded that this type of therapy favourably affects development of motor functions in children. They examined 511 children and their results were compared after 6 months and then again after 18 months. They found a statistically significant difference ($p = 0.035$) in the improved motor skills in the children taking part in the DAT sessions [10].

A review of the effects of other therapies on the psychomotor development of children with intellectual disability suggests that Dog-Assisted Therapy evaluated in the present study leads to comparable positive outcomes. For example, Ferreira et al. analysed the effects of a psychomotor intervention from the perspective of sensorial integration in children with intellectual disability. The study group included children aged 5 to 12 years. The therapy was designed to include physical education, described as "psychomotor education/reeducation", and comprised 44 sessions, 50 min each. The findings showed that the program affected the following psychomotor domains: Body schema, tonicity, laterality, as well as global and final praxis. Less visible effects were identified in balance and space-time structure [46]. Similar effects were identified in the current study. Furthermore, Lucas et al. carried out a systematic review with meta-analysis to examine effects of conservative therapies designed to improve gross motor skills in children with various neurodevelopmental disorders. Nine articles met inclusion criteria. The authors reported that some task-oriented interventions can effectively be used for the above purpose [47]. On the other hand, Wuang et al. in quasi-experimental controlled study investigated effectiveness of sensory integrative therapy, perceptual-motor approach, and neurodevelopmental treatment in children with mild intellectual disability. The three types of interventions were applied to 120 children randomly assigned to three specific subgroups. Assessments performed with measures of sensorimotor function carried out after the interventions showed significantly better scores in the treatment groups compared to the controls (receiving no treatment) on almost all measures. Sensory integrative therapy more visibly affected fine motor skills, upper-limb coordination, and sensory integration. Perceptual-motor therapy produced significant gains in the children's gross motor skills, while the neurodevelopmental treatment resulted in the smallest changes in most measures taken into account [48]. Conversely, Bukhovets and Romanchuk assessed effects of Bobath therapy on psychomotor development in children aged 3–6 years, presenting with organic central nervous system involvement. The study was designed to evaluate the children's psychophysical state before and after neurodevelopmental treatment continued for 10 days in hospital. The findings showed a positive dynamics of motor activity and motor skills learning, which confirms the effectiveness of Bobath therapy as a method supporting psychomotor development of children aged 3–6 years with organic lesions in the central nervous system [49]. These observations are not consistent with the findings reported by Zanon et al. who published a systematic review following the recommendations of the Cochrane Handbook for Systematic Reviews of Interventions to assess the effects of neurodevelopmental treatment (Bobath) for children with cerebral palsy. They performed a comprehensive search for clinical trials designed to assess Bobath method in comparison to conventional physical therapy applied to children with cerebral palsy and identified three randomized clinical trials involving 66 children. The analyses showed that effectiveness of neurodevelopmental treatment and conventional physical therapy did not differ in the case of gross motor function [50]. In summary, it may be concluded that sensorimotor approaches should be selected taking into account specific needs of a child because each approach may present advantages with regard to certain aspects of sensorimotor functions.

The current analyses did not identify between-group differences at the end of the therapy program (i.e., after 10 months), however the DAT Group achieved significantly better scores in postural imitation and finger identification tests, compared to the controls, at the follow-up exam two months after the therapy was completed, which may reflect delayed improvement attributable to the DAT. This may be associated with the fact that the follow-up exam was performed at the end of the summer holidays. Typically, during a break from the day care facility children spend more time at home where they do not receive any specialised therapy. In fact, we interviewed the parents to find out whether their children had participated in additional therapeutic activities in the summer. No parents reported that their children had received any form of therapy in that period. We cannot rule out, with absolute certainty, that some external factors indeed impacted the final results. It can, however, be speculated that the functions stimulated by the DAT therapy were more extensively (and freely) practiced in home setting which possibly provides more opportunities for a variety of independently performed activities, compared to a day care centre where activities are generally more structured. This may have led to the children's increased confidence in the use of the newly acquired abilities. In other words, it could be suggested that the 10-month period of the DAT, which involved exposition of the children to the stimuli, was more of a preliminary (theoretical) training, while the summer break associated with a change of the environment provided room for independent practical training of the skills. It is possible this period of "extra practice" enabled the children from the DAT group to gain greater self-reliance in the activities of daily living, which was eventually reflected by better scores acquired during the follow-up tests, compared to the controls.

In summary, the brief literature review above shows that most studies report positive results; DAT favourably affects the patients subjected to such interventions. Hence, it may be postulated that DAT is a good way to promote the process of rehabilitation, which is also supported by the current findings. However, it is necessary to continue the related research in larger groups of subjects and to apply different research tools.

The strength of this study is linked with the fact that the analysis of the long-term effects of the therapy program is based on three assessments. Functional implications of this study are related to the fact that the acquired results may be of importance for clinical practice since they present evidence confirming long-term effectiveness of DAT and constitute an encouragement for introducing DAT as a supplementary method, which may be applied along with conventional therapies in children with mild intellectual disability in facilities providing treatment to this population.

Study Limitations

The findings of the current study apply only to children with mild intellectual disability. It is necessary to continue research and investigate the effects of DAT related to psychomotor efficiency of children with moderate and severe intellectual disability. Another limitation of the study is linked with the low number of participants. In the case of small samples, there is a greater risk that the results may be unreliable; besides, in small samples, statistical significance is found less frequently. As a rule, it is assumed that the larger the sample, the easier it is to detect any changes. Further research should involve a larger group of children with intellectual disability, and it would also be worthwhile to investigate impact of other factors such as age and sex on effectiveness of DAT.

5. Conclusions

The study showed certain long-term effects of dog-assisted therapy in the functioning of children with mild intellectual disabilities, aged 10–13 years. The results achieved by the children in the DAT group in some cases were significantly improved, as reflected by measurements performed over time. There were no significant differences in the baseline results and in the tests performed at the end of the therapy program between the children in the DAT group and the controls. Ultimately, however, at the two-month follow-up, the DAT group achieved better results than the controls in motor planning (postural imitation test) and in the sense of touch, attention, and concentration (finger identification test). Despite the fact that the measurement performed at the end of the therapy did not show significant differences between the DAT group and the controls, the results acquired at the two-month follow-up reflected long-term gains in the treatment group in the domain of motor planning (postural imitation test). Our findings suggest that dog-assisted interventions may effectively be used as a complementary treatment in children with physical and mental disability. The acquired results may be of importance for clinical practice since they present evidence confirming long-term effectiveness of DAT and constitute an encouragement for introducing DAT as a supplementary method, which may be applied along with conventional therapies in children with mild intellectual disability in facilities providing treatment to this population. This fact should be taken into account by those designing therapeutic programs in facilities providing treatment to this population of children.

Author Contributions: A.W.-N.: conceptualized and designed the study, performed the research study; wrote the main manuscript, and approved the final manuscript as submitted.; A.G.: conceptualized and designed the study, carried out the formal analysis, wrote a major part of the manuscript, supervised, and approved the final manuscript as submitted; J.D.: performed the research study, drafted the initial manuscript; B.P., M.D.: performed the statistical analysis, critically reviewed the manuscript. All authors have read and agreed to the published version of the manuscript.

Funding: This research received no external funding.

Institutional Review Board Statement: The study was conducted according to the guidelines of the Declaration of Helsinki, and approved by the Ethics Committee Commission of the Medical Faculty (4 February 2017).

Informed Consent Statement: Informed consent was obtained from all subjects involved in the study.

Data Availability Statement: Data available in a publicly accessible repository.

Conflicts of Interest: The authors declare no conflict of interest.

References

1. Widmar, D.H.; Feuillan, K.A. Animal-assisted therapy. In *Physical Medicine and Rehabilitation—The Complete Approach*; Grabois, M., Garrison, S.J., Hart, K.A., Lehmkuhl, L.D., Eds.; Blackwell: Oxford, UK, 2000; Volume 733, p. 61.
2. Maber-Aleksandrowicz, S.; Avent, C.; Hassiotis, A. A systematic review of animal-assisted therapy on psychosocial outcomes in people with intellectual disability. *Res. Dev. Disabil.* **2016**, *49–50*, 322–338. [CrossRef] [PubMed]
3. Silkwood-Sherer, D.J.; Killian, C.B.; Long, T.M.; Martin, K.S. Hip-potherapy—An intervention to habilitate balance deficits in children with movement disorders: A clinical trial. *Phys. Ther.* **2012**, *92*, 17–707. [CrossRef] [PubMed]
4. Tseng, S.H.; Cheng, H.C.; Tam, K.W. Systematic review and meta-analysis of the effect of equine assisted activities and therapies on gross motor outcome in children with cerebral palsy. *Disabil. Rehabil.* **2013**, *35*, 89–99. [CrossRef] [PubMed]
5. Zadnikar, M.; Kastrin, A. Effects of hippotherapy and therapeutic horseback riding on postural control or balance in children with cerebral palsy:a meta-analysis. *Dev. Med. Child Neurol.* **2011**, *53*, 684–691. [CrossRef]

6. Schuck, S.E.B.; Emmerson, N.A.; Fine, A.H.; Lakes, K.D. Canine-assisted therapy for children with ADHD: Preliminary findings from the Positive Assertive Cooperative Kids study. *J. Attent. Disor.* **2015**, *19*, 125–137. [CrossRef]
7. Kwon, J.Y.; Chang, H.J.; Lee, J.Y.; Ha, Y.; Lee, P.K.; Kim, Y.H. Effects of hippotherapy on gait parameters in children with bilateral spastic cerebral palsy. *Arch. Phys. Med. Rehabil.* **2011**, *92*, 774–779. [CrossRef]
8. Lundqvist, M.; Carlsson, P.; Sjödahl, R.; Theodorsson, E.; Levin, L.Å. Patient benefit of dog-assisted interventions in health care: A systematic review. *BMC Complementary Altern. Med.* **2017**, *17*, 358. [CrossRef]
9. Muñoz Lasaa, S.; Máximo Bocanegrab, N.; Valero Alcaidea, R. Animal assisted interventions in neurorehabilitation: A review of the most recent literature. *Neurology* **2015**, *30*, 1–7. [CrossRef]
10. Piek, J.P.; McLaren, S.; Kane, R.; Jensen, L.; Dender, A.; Roberts, C.; Rooney, R.; Packer, T.; Straker, L. Does the Animal Fun program improve motor performance in children aged 4–6 years? *Hum. Mov. Sci.* **2013**, *32*, 1086–1096. [CrossRef]
11. Jorge, A.; Rigoli, D.; Kane, R.; Melaren, S. Does Animal Fun improve aiming and catching and balance skills in youn children. *Res. Dev. Disabil.* **2019**, *84*, 122–130.
12. Richeson, N. Effects of animal-assisted therapy on agitated behaviors and social interactions of older adults with dementia. *Am. J. Alzheimers Dis. Other Demen.* **2003**, *18*, 353–358. [CrossRef] [PubMed]
13. Kongable, L.G.; Buckwalter, K.C.; Stolley, J.M. The effects of pet therapy on the social behavior of institutionalized Alzheimer's clients. *Arch. Psychiatr. Nurse* **1989**, *3*, 191–198.
14. Scorzato, I.; Zaninotto, L.; Chiara, M.; Cavedon, L. Effects of Dog-Assisted Therapy on Comunication and Basic Social Skills of Adults with Intellectual Disabilities: A piot Study. *Intellectal Dev. Disabil.* **2017**, *55*, 125–139. [CrossRef] [PubMed]
15. Gochewa, V.; Hund-Georgiadis, M.; Hediger, K. Effects of animal assisted therapy on concentration and attention span in patients with acquired brain injury: A randomized controlled trial. *Neuropsychology* **2018**, *32*, 54–64. [CrossRef] [PubMed]
16. McCullough, A.; Ruehrdanz, A.; Jenkins, M.A.; Gilmer, M.J.; Olson, J.; Pawar, A.; Holley, L.; Sierra-Rivera, S.; Linder, D.E.; Pichette, D.; et al. Measuring the Effects of an Animal-Assisted Intervention for Pediatric Oncology Patients and Their Parents: A Multisite Randomized Controlled Trial. *J. Pediatr. Oncol. Nurs.* **2018**, *35*, 159–177. [CrossRef] [PubMed]
17. Muela, A.; Balluerka, N.; Amiano, N.; Caldentey, M.A.; Aliri, J. Animal-assisted psychotherapy for young people with behavioural problems in residential care. *Clin. Psychol. Psychother.* **2017**, *24*, O1485–O1494. [CrossRef]
18. Schuck, S.E.; Johnson, H.L.; Abdullah, M.M.; Stehli, A.; Fine, A.H.; Lakes, K.D. The Role of Animal Assisted Intervention on Improving Self-Esteem in Children with Attention Deficit/Hyperactivity Disorder. *Front. Pediatr.* **2018**, *6*, 300. [CrossRef]
19. Hill, J.; Ziviani, J.; Driscoll, C.; Cawdell-Smith, J. Can Canine-Assisted Interventions Affect the Social Behaviours of Children on the Autism Spectrum? *Rev. J. Autism. Dev. Disord.* **2019**, *6*, 13–25. [CrossRef]
20. Boguszewski, D.; Świderska, B.; Adamczyk, J.G.; Białoszewski, D. Evaluation of the effectiveness of the dog-assisted therapy in the rehabilitation of children with Down syndrome. *Prelim. Rep. Eur. J. Clin. Exp. Med.* **2013**, *2*, 194–202.
21. Drwięga, G.; Pietruczuk, Z. Dog therapy as a form of supporting the development of a disabled child. *Niepełnosprawność Zagadnienia Probl. Rozw.* **2015**, *3*, 57–68.
22. Grandgeorge, M.; Hausberger, M. Human-animal relationships: From daily life to animal-assisted therapies. *Ann. Dell' Inst. Super. Sanita* **2011**, *47*, 397–408.
23. Friedmann, E.; Katcher, A.H.; Lynch, J.J.; Thomas, S.A. Animal companions and one-year survival of patients after discharge from a coronary care unit. *Public Health Rep.* **1980**, *95*, 307–312. [PubMed]
24. De Rose, P.; Cannas, E.; Cantiello, P.R. Donkey-assisted rehabilitation program for children: A pilot study. *Ann. Dell' Inst. Super. Sanita* **2011**, *47*, 391–396.
25. Ballarini, G. Pet therapy. Animals in human therapy. *Acta Biol. Med.* **2003**, *74*, 97–100.
26. Keith, T.Z.; Fine, J.G.; Taub, G.E.; Reynolds, M.R.; Kranzler, J.H. Higher order, multisample, confirmatory factor analysis of the Wechsler Intelligence Scale for Children–Fourth Edition: What does it measure? *Sch. Psychol. Rev.* **2006**, *35*, 108–127. [CrossRef]

27. Hrabok, M.; Brooks, B.L.; Fay-McClymont, T.B.; Sherman, E.M.S. Wechsler Intelligence Scale for Children-Fourth Edition (WISC-IV) Short-form validity: A comparison study in pediatric epilepsy. *Child. Neuropsychol.* **2012**, *20*, 49–59. [CrossRef] [PubMed]
28. Suresh, K. An overview of randomization techniques: An unbiased assessment of outcome in clinical research. *J. Hum. Reprod Sci.* **2011**, *4*, 8–11. [CrossRef]
29. Grewelf, F. The Bourdon-Wiersma test. *Folia Psychiatr. Neurol. Psychiatr.* **1953**, *56*, 694–703.
30. Ayres, A.J. *Sensory Integration and the Child*, 2nd ed.; Western Psychological Services: Los Angeles, CA, USA, 2004.
31. Kilroy, E.; Aziz-Zadeh, L.; Cermak, S. Ayres theories of autism and sensory integration revisited: What contemporary neuroscience has to say. *Brain Sci.* **2019**, *9*, 68. [CrossRef]
32. Czenczek-Lewandowska, E.; Leszczak, J.; Baran, J.; Weres, A.; Wyszyńska, J.; Lewandowski, B.; Dąbrowski, M.; Mazur, A. Levels of Physical Activity in Children and Adolescents with Type 1 Diabetes in Relation to the Healthy Comparators and to the Method of Insulin Therapy Used. *Int. J. Environ. Res. Public Health* **2019**, *16*, 3498. [CrossRef]
33. Guzik, A.; Drużbicki, M.; Kwolek, A.; Przysada, G.; Bazarnik-Mucha, K.; Szczepanik, M.; Wolan-Nieroda, A.; Sobolewski, M. The paediatric version of Wisconsin gait scale, adaptation for children with hemiplegic cerebral palsy: A prospective observational study. *BMC Pediatr.* **2018**, *18*, 301. [CrossRef] [PubMed]
34. Rusek, W.; Leszczak, J.; Baran, J.; Adamczyk, M.; Weres, A.; Baran, R.; Inglot, G.; Czenczek-Lewandowska, E.; Porada, S.; Pop, T. Role of body mass category in the development of faulty postures in school-age children from a rural area in south-eastern Poland: A cross-sectional study. *BMJ Open* **2019**, *9*. [CrossRef] [PubMed]
35. Baran, J.; Weres, A.; Czenczek-Lewandowska, E.; Leszczak, J.; Kalandyk-Osinko, K.; Łuszczki, E.; Sobek, G.; Mazur, A. Excessive Gestational Weight Gain: Long-Term Consequences for the Child. *J. Clin. Med.* **2020**, *9*, 3795. [CrossRef] [PubMed]
36. Dilek, T.E.; Sibel, C. Dog-assisted therapies and activities in rehabilitation of children with cerebral palsy and physical and mental disabilities. *Int. J. Environ. Res. Public Health* **2015**, *12*, 5046–5060.
37. Fung, S.; Leung, A. Pilot Study Investigating the Role of Therapy Dogs in Facilitating Social Interaction among Children with Autism. *J. Contemp. Psychother.* **2014**, *44*, 253–262. [CrossRef]
38. François, M.; Jennifer, F. Animal-Assisted Therapy for Children with Pervasive Developmental Disorders. *West. J. Nurs. Res.* **2002**, *24*, 657–670.
39. Bülent, E.; Hlya, K.; Irem, D. Sensory integration and activities of daily living in children with developmental coordination disorder. *Ital. J. Pediatr.* **2012**, *38*, 14. [CrossRef]
40. Schoemaker, M.M.; Wees, V.; Flapper, B.; Verheij-Jansen, N.; Scholten Jaegers, S.; Geuze, R.H. Perceptual skills of children with developmental coordination disorder. *Hum. Mov. Sci.* **2001**, *20*, 111–133. [CrossRef]
41. Reed, R.; Ferrer, L.; Villegas, N. Natural healers: A review of animal assisted therapy and activities as complementary treatment for chronic conditions. *Rev. Lat. Am. Enferm.* **2012**, *20*, 612–618. [CrossRef]
42. Nawrocka-Rohnka, J. Dogtherapy as a method of supporting rehabilitation for child with disorder of development. *Med. News* **2010**, *79*, 304–310.
43. Gee, N.R.; Harris, S.L.; Johnson, K.L. The role of therapy dogs in speed and accuracy to complete motor skills tasks for preschool children. *Anthrozoos A Multidiscip. J. Interact. People Anim.* **2007**, *20*, 375–386. [CrossRef]
44. Bunker, L.K. The role of play and motor skill development in building children's selfconfidence and self-esteem. *Elem. Sch. J. Spec. Issue Sports Phys. Educ.* **1991**, *91*, 467–471.
45. Macauley, B. Animal-assisted therapy for persons with aphasia: A pilot study. *J. Rehabil. Res. Dev.* **2006**, *43*, 357–366. [CrossRef] [PubMed]
46. Ferreira, E.F.; Teixeira, F.A.C.; Pereira, T.E. Sensorial Integration and Intellectual Disabilities: Influence of Psychomotor Intervention. *IOSR J. Sports Phys. Educ.* **2016**, *3*, 44–49.
47. Lucas, B.R.; Elliott, E.J.; Coggan, S.; Pinto, R.Z.; Jirikowic, T.; McCoy, S.W.; Latimer, J. Interventions to improve gross motor performance in children with neurodevelopmental disorders: A meta-analysis. *BMC Pediatr.* **2016**, *16*, 193. [CrossRef]
48. Wuang, Y.P.; Wang, C.C.; Huang, M.H.; Su, C.Y. Prospective study of the effect of sensory integration, neurodevelopmental treatment, and perceptual-motor therapy on the sensorimotor performance in children with mild mental retardation. *Am. J. Occup.* **2009**, *63*, 441–452. [CrossRef]
49. Bukhovets, B.O.; Romanchuk, A.P. Bobath therapy in correction of psychomotor development of children with organic injuries CNS. *J. Health Sci.* **2014**, *4*, 71–78.

50. Zanon, M.A.; Pacheco, R.L.; Latorraca, C.O.C.; Martimbianco, A.L.C.; Pachito, D.V.; Riera, R. Neurodevelopmental Treatment (Bobath) for Children With Cerebral Palsy: A Systematic Review. *J. Child. Neurol.* **2019**, *34*, 679–686. [CrossRef]

Publisher's Note: MDPI stays neutral with regard to jurisdictional claims in published maps and institutional affiliations.

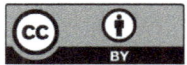

© 2020 by the authors. Licensee MDPI, Basel, Switzerland. This article is an open access article distributed under the terms and conditions of the Creative Commons Attribution (CC BY) license (http://creativecommons.org/licenses/by/4.0/).

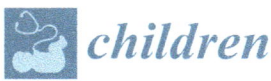

Article

Weighted Blankets and Sleep Quality in Children with Autism Spectrum Disorders: A Single-Subject Design

Bryan M. Gee [1,*], Kimberly Lloyd [2], Jesse Sutton [3] and Tyler McOmber [4]

1. College of Rehabilitation Sciences, Rocky Mountain University of Health Professions, Provo, UT 84606, USA
2. School of Rehabilitation and Communication Sciences, Idaho State University, Pocatello, ID 83209, USA; lloykim3@isu.edu
3. Mary Lanning Healthcare, Hastings, NE 68901, USA; jessesutton.38@gmail.com
4. Idaho Home Health and Hospice, Gooding, ID 83330, USA; tcmcomber@gmail.com
* Correspondence: bryan.gee@rm.edu

Received: 11 November 2020; Accepted: 24 December 2020; Published: 27 December 2020

Abstract: The purpose of the study was to explore the efficacy of weighted blanket applications and sleep quality in children with autism spectrum disorder and behavioral manifestations of sensory processing deficits. Two 4-year-old participants diagnosed with autism spectrum disorder who also experienced sleep disturbances took part in a single-subject design study. Objective sleep measures and caregiver surveys were tracked for a baseline period of eight days, followed by a 14-day weighted blanket intervention and a seven-day withdrawal phase. Caregiver reports and objective data were evaluated using visual analysis and the percentage of non-overlapping data methods. The results suggest minimal changes in sleep patterns as a result of the weighted blanket intervention. The findings based on using a weighted blanket intervention were enhanced morning mood after night use and a significantly decreased time to fall asleep for participants, though they were not strong enough to recommend for clinical use. Future directions include single-subject and cohort-designed studies exploring the efficacy of weighted blankets with increasing sleep quality among children with autism.

Keywords: weighted blankets; sensory-based interventions; autism spectrum disorder

1. Introduction

Autism is a complex neurodevelopmental condition with hallmark features that include atypical language and communication skills, poor social interaction, impaired executive functioning, sensory processing, and motor skill coordination [1]. The condition presents with comorbid psychiatric and medical conditions which may include anxiety disorder, oppositional defiant disorder, attention-deficit/hyperactivity disorder, intellectual disability, immune system irregularities, gastrointestinal disorder, sleep disturbances and epilepsy and seizure disorder [2]. As mentioned with the medical conditions, are sleep disturbances and low sleep quality [3] is the focus of this paper. Research estimates that 44% to 83% of individuals (adults and children) with autism experience sleep disturbances [4]. Humphreys et al. [5] reported a reduced sleep duration of 17 to 43 min in children (30 months to 11 years) with autism as compared to children without autism.

Additionally, children (18 to 42 months) with autism have impaired sleep patterns [5]. Sleep duration are shortened in children with autism due to later bedtimes, earlier risings, and frequent wakings (three or more wakings a night) [5]. Malow et al. [6] found that those children with autism who slept poorly showed a decrease in rapid eye movement (REM) sleep and an increase in non-rapid eye movement (NREM) sleep stage 4. Malow et al. [6] also reported that children with autism who have a sleep disorder show an exacerbation of behavioral challenges throughout the next day. Children with autism can have sleep impairments, which can adversely affect their quality of life with an increase in aggressive behavior, anxiety, increased parental stress, and family life quality [7].

Further confounding the issue is the prevalence of sensory processing disturbances among children with autism has upon activities of daily living, particularly sleep. A systematic review conducted by Ismael et al. [8] reported that the majority children with autism experience sensory disturbances that impact sleep, primarily in the domain of sensory avoiding or sensory over responsivity. In a study using behavioral and physiological measures, Reynolds et al. [9] found that children aged six to 12 years with autism have a higher prevalence of atypical sensory behaviors (sensory under responsiveness and over responsiveness) and sleep disturbances than typical children of the same age.

Commonly used interventions to support sleep quality among children with autism include pharmacological agents [10], behavioral and contextual sleep hygiene changes [8], caregiver education, and training [11]. However, an intervention that has seen increased use in attempting to improve sleep quality among children with autism is a weighted blanket [12].

Weighted blankets are used as an intervention strategy to improve sleep in children with autism who have sleep impairments [12,13]. The current underlying posit for weighted blanket use is to provide deep touch pressure stimuli, thus acting as a calming mediator by increasing parasympathetic activity [13,14]. The mediating intervention in the blanket is weight imbedded into the blanket primarily through plastic beads or balls to approximately 10% of the user's body weight [12–16]. The weight is either modified through pouches and pockets with interchangeable weights or are more permanent with non-modifiable weight. Weighted blankets are passive sensory-based adjunctive intervention that is applied to a child or adult to reduce unwanted behaviors rooted in sensory modulation impairments [12,13]. Some authors state that weighted blankets help individuals stabilize and modulate sensory input and lower anxiety during stressful situations by enhancing parasympathetic activation [17,18].

Reviewing the literature related to sensory processing and children without a neurological or behavioral impairment (including children with autism) yielded some sparse resources. Foitzik and Brown [19] reported that typically developing school-aged children who demonstrate sensory disturbances with tactile sensory processing (hyporesponsive) slept longer and had fewer night wakings. Furthermore, Fiotzik and Brown [19] reported that children and adults demonstrate fewer sleep quality disturbances in conjunction with more typical sensory processing patterns than those with sensory processing related behaviors [19]. Vriend et al. [20] reported that children with low sleep quality may demonstrate difficulty in sensory processing domains, specifically emotional regulation. In a study of sensory processing and sleep among infants and toddlers, Vasak et al. [21] reported correlations between increased sensory seeking behaviors and shorter daytime sleep duration (naps). Such correlations also applied to increased sensory sensitivity behaviors and increased time to fall asleep (at night). In school-aged children diagnosed with attention deficit hyperactivity disorder (ADHD), Shochat, Tzischinsky, and Engel-Yeager [22] reported that children with ADHD experienced disturbances with sleep quality in part due to tactile sensory over-responsivity (SOR).

While sleep disturbances are commonplace in children with autism, minimal empirical evidence exists examining potential interventions to enhance sleep quality using sensory-based interventions [12]. Parents and caregivers often seek strategies to increase sleep quality and duration for their children with autism [12]. Some of the literature in occupational therapy has described applying sensory-based intervention to influence a child's level of arousal, behavioral organization, and on-task behavior [15]. One potential sensory-based strategy to enhance sleep patterns in children with autism is the use of a weighted blanket [15].

Sensory integration theory [22,23] posits that deep pressure sensory stimulation (touch) may create calming effects as a result of the modulation (control) of the central nervous system. Specifically, deep pressure touch influences reticular formation activity and autonomic nervous system function [20]. Authors postulate that deep pressure touch provided via weighted blankets offers a feeling of safety, comfort, and groundedness [12]. In some cases, weighted blankets are used to help individuals stabilize and modulate responsiveness to sensory input in order to lower anxiety [12,17,18], level of arousal, decrease impulsivity, increase attention to task, and decrease maladaptive internalizing emotions [12,13].

Sensory integration theory also accounts for varying types of sensory responsivity. Schaaf and Anzalone [24] describe sensory responsivity as the ability to receive, organize, and interpret sensory stimuli across multiple sensory domains/systems including oral, visual, tactile, vestibular, proprioceptive, auditory, and interoception. Therefore, sensory responsivity is "the ability to regulate the response to sensory input" ([23], p. 277). Sensory over-responsivity (SOR) is a subtype of sensory processing disorder where the child or individual responds to a cluster of sensations in an extreme or exaggerated manner [23]. Reynolds, Lane, and Mullen [9] found that children with autism and SOR had more difficulties with sleep than children with only autism. Shochat, Tzischinsky, and Engel-Yeger [22] and Vasak, Williamson, Garden, and Zwiker [21] hypothesized that increased sleep disturbances might be associated with increased sensory sensitivity due to a low neurological threshold and use of a passive self-regulation strategy. Vasak and colleagues [21] also reported that infants and toddlers demonstrating increased sensory sensitivity required a longer time to settle to fall sleep. Evidence exists that links patterns of similar sensory sensitivities with restless behavior and difficulty falling asleep among typical school-aged children and adults [22].

Studies of weighted blanket interventions for children with autism are emerging in the literature. Gringras and colleagues [14] conducted a study with 73 children ages 5–16 with autism who had a concomitant report of a caregiver's sleep disturbance in the previous five months. The authors implemented a crossover design toggling weighted blanket application for two weeks with a non-weighted blanket. The primary outcome was total sleep time as measured by an actigraph (a wearable device like a watch that continuously measures sleep parameters). Gringras and colleagues' [14] primary finding for children with a wide range of autism severity levels were that weighted blankets were not any more effective than a typical blanket in helping children with autism improve their total sleep quantity.

Despite the lack of significant findings related to weighted blankets improving sleep quality among children with autism, Gringras and colleagues [14] reported that parent's/participant's experienced an improvement in next-day behaviors captured using a sleep diary kept by the participants' parents/caregivers. Gringras and colleagues [14] hypothesized that an improvement in next day behaviors might have been due to improved bedtime behaviors (i.e., routines). Research design aspects that may have improved overall parent/child interactions include parents wishing to please the study team, or parents observed improvements that the objective measures were not sensitive enough to capture.

Gee and colleagues [15,16] implemented a weighted blanket intervention using a single-subject ABA design in two separate studies. They found minimal changes in sleep duration and morning mood via caregiver report. Gee and colleagues [15,16] examined whether weighted blankets have positively impacted time to fall asleep, the number of wakings, duration of sleep, and morning mood for two children with autism and SOR. Using visual analysis of caregivers' perceptions, the overall findings demonstrated minimal improvement of the measured constructs related to sleep quality. Participants exhibited evidence of an increase in the total amount of sleep per night and a slight decrease in time to fall asleep. However, morning mood did not consistently improve with the weighted blanket's use across all participants [15,16].

Finally, a systematic review [25] was conducted evaluating general effectiveness of weighted blankets across various population conditions. The authors concluded that weighted blankets might be an appropriate therapeutic tool in reducing anxiety; however, the authors indicated that more evidence is needed to recommend their use in improving sleep quality among diverse populations.

A paucity of research exists exploring the efficacy of weighted blanket interventions with younger children with autism (e.g., three to six years old), SOR to tactile and auditory stimulus, and sleep disturbances. Therefore, the present study's primary aim was to examine weighted blankets in younger children with autism, SOR (tactile and auditory sensory domains), and sleep disturbances (difficulty falling asleep, staying asleep, and poor morning mood). A secondary aim was to use intervention and measurement tools commonly utilized in occupational therapy practice and affordable to clinical professionals (e.g., weighted blankets and Sense Sleep App) and caregivers (e.g., weighted blanket).

Research Question

Does a weighted blanket impact sleep quality among children with autism, sleep disturbances, and sensory over-responsivity?

2. Materials and Methods

The current study implemented an ABA research design with pre- and post-test phases [26]. The research design was selected based upon the alignment of the purpose and research question guiding the study. Further, the design is used due to the low availability of a clinical sample in a largely rural and medically underserved area in the Intermountain West region of the United States. The overall study aimed at increasing the duration of the intervention phase, using a caregiver questionnaire tracking participant behavioral changes and using a sample of younger children that were implemented in the Gringras et al. [14] and Gee et al. [15,16] studies.

The pre-test phase consisted of participants' caregivers completing subjective measures related to their child's sleep behavior patterns and sensory processing preferences/challenges. The Sensory Processing Measure–Preschool version (SPM-P) [27] and Children's Sleep Habits Questionnaire (CSHQ) [28] were administered to ensure the participant met the study's inclusion criteria. The SPM-P is a judgment-based rating scale to measure distinct sensory processing patterns (tactile, vestibular, auditory, visual, etc.), praxis, and social participation among preschool-aged children (3–5 years of age). The CSHQ is a judgment-based rating scale completed by caregivers to measure sleep habits in children ages 4 to 10. The measure has an internal consistency of 0.78 with a sensitivity of 0.80. The classification accuracy of sleep disorders among the targeted age range is 80% [27].

The first phase of the study labeled the baseline phase, lasted for at least seven days. During the baseline phase, the participants' caregivers completed a five-question, non-standardized Daily Caregiver Survey that quantitatively identified the time to fall asleep at night, duration of night sleep, number of times the child woke up during the night, and a child's morning mood. The survey was developed as an attempt to integrate recommendations from the Gringras et al. study [14]. After completing the baseline measures, the participants transitioned to a 14-day weighted blanket intervention phase. Throughout the intervention phase, participants slept with a weighted blanket, and the caregivers continued to complete the daily surveys. After completing the intervention phase, the weighted blankets were withdrawn, and the study transitioned into the withdrawal phase. During the withdrawal phase, caregivers continued to complete daily surveys for eight days.

2.1. Method of Recruitment

The Human Subjects Committee approved the study at Idaho State University (Pocatello, ID) (on 10 February 2017, IRB-FY2016-170). Study participants were recruited via brochures distributed by the first author and primary investigator (PI) to local pediatricians, pediatric occupational therapists, and speech-language pathologists. Interested caregivers contacted the PI directly to receive additional study details and ask questions. During the initial phone conversation, the PI asked several questions to determine eligibility (see inclusion criteria). If the participant met the inclusion criteria and demonstrated a willingness to participate in the study, written informed consent was obtained. Informed consent was obtained before the participants beginning the study.

2.2. Inclusion Criteria

Study participants were required to meet the following inclusion criteria to participate in this study. The child needed to:

(1) have a medical diagnosis (provided by the caregiver and treating physician) of autism;
(2) demonstrate the behavioral manifestations of sensory over-responsivity (T-score of 70 or higher on the tactile and/or auditory domains on the SPM-P) [27];
(3) qualitative ratings of "usually" (5 days per week) or higher in multiple aspects of sleep quality on the CSHQ [28];
(4) be between the ages of three and six.

The caregiver needed to:

(1) be able to report if the child had difficulty falling asleep and staying asleep,
(2) speak and understand the English language;
(3) have daily access to a reliable internet connection during the study period;
(4) be able to complete an online Daily Caregiver Survey for 30 days;
(5) be able to implement a weighted blanket as part of the child's sleep routine for 14 consecutive days.

Participants and caregivers were excluded from the study if they did not meet the above-listed inclusion criteria.

Description of the Participants

Participant one, using the pseudonym John, was a four-year, five-month-old male child with a reported autism diagnosis that included a cognitive impairment. The findings from the SPM-P [27] caregiver report screener indicated a Definite Dysfunction in the behavioral manifestations of over-responsivity to tactile (T-Score of 72), auditory (T-Score of 78), and visual sensory (T-Score of 70) stimuli. The qualitative results from the CSHQ [28] caregiver report ratings indicated he demonstrated poor sleep quality as evidenced by difficulty falling asleep ("always"—seven days a week), staying asleep ("always"—seven days a week), wakes up too early ("usually"—five days a week) and experiences a poor morning mood ("usually"—five days a week). No other medical comorbidities were reported.

Participant two using the pseudonym Katie, was a four year, one-month-old female child with a reported diagnosis of autism. The findings from the SPM-P [28] caregiver report screener indicated a Definite Dysfunction in the behavioral manifestations of over-responsivity to tactile (T-Score of 80), auditory (T-Score of 74), and visual sensory (T-Score of 73) stimuli. The qualitative results from the CSHQ caregiver report ratings indicated that she demonstrated difficulty staying asleep (wakes more than once at night ("usually"—five days a week)), wakes up too early ("always"—seven days a week) and experiences a poor morning mood ("usually"—five days a week). No other medical comorbidities were reported.

2.3. Dependent Variables

Daily Caregiver Surveys (delivered online via SurveyMonkey®) were completed throughout all study phases. The non-standardized survey consisted of six subjective questions assessing the participants' sleep habits from the previous day and mood the morning the survey was completed. Each survey was completed by the caregiver based upon their best recollection of the previous night's events. The survey tracked the caregivers' perception of their child's sleep latency, number of naps, duration of naps, number of night wakings, sleep duration, and morning mood. Morning mood was operationalized as feelings, varying in intensity and duration, and usually involving more than one emotion [29]. In this case, the authors identified agitation/calm as one emotion related to mood. The assessment of morning mood (i.e., agitation/calm) allowed for the participants' caregivers to rate the current level of the child's agitation compared to the prior day using a five-point Likert like scale (more agitated, slightly more agitated, no difference, slightly calmer, and more calm).

The Sense [30] Sleep App was used to objectively track variables, including the participant's overall sleep quality, total hours of sleep, and the number of hours of deep sleep. The Sense Sleep App included a motion tracker called a "pill" attached to the participants' pillowcase or sheet at the head of the bed. The tracker's base component sat next to the bed and captured movement-related information from the pill attached to the participant's pillow or sheet. The Sense Sleep App exported data that were transmitted and stored from the pill and the base each morning to an Apple Inc. device (e.g., iPad provided by the PI to each participant). Upon return of the iPad at the end of the research study, the data were transferred to a Microsoft Excel spreadsheet. This commercially purchased device had not been utilized in any peer-reviewed literature. Due to the proprietary nature of the device, information related to reliability and validity were unavailable. From a pragmatic perspective, the Sense Sleep App was used because it was a non-wearable system. The target population is young children (3–6 years old) who also demonstrated tactile sensory over-responsivity, which removed the option of using wearable devices such as the Garmin Jr. HR. Additionally, the cost was approximately USD 99.00, which is affordable for most clinicians to utilize in practice.

2.4. Intervention

During the intervention phase of the study, participants used weighted blankets for 14 consecutive nights. These weighted blankets were the SensaCalm® brand, custom made, and were provided by the PI. The weighted blankets were designed to be 10% of each child's body weight adhering to the prototypical weighted blanket protocol [13–16]. The SensaCalm® blankets used for the study ranged from 3–7 pounds to accommodate the varying weights of potential participants and ranged between USD 40.00 and 80.00. The blanket brand was chosen based upon the affordable cost, durability, equal distribution of weight across the blanket. When the weighted blankets were provided, caregivers were given instructions on safely and effectively using them. Caregivers were instructed to only use the blankets at night (i.e., not during nap time or quiet time); only use the blanket if the child was able to remove it on their own; cover the child's body, arms, and feet but not their head or face; check on the child occasionally while using the blanket; adjust other bedding while using the weighted blanket to ensure the child was not too hot, and to contact the PI if the weighted blanket was showing signs of wear. Additionally, caregivers of the participants reported that they slept in their own bed (as opposed to the caregivers, or another location) through this study's duration.

2.5. Method of Analysis

Data were analyzed through visual analysis of repeated measure graphs generated using Microsoft Excel, version 16, as described by Kennedy [31]. Visual analysis is widely accepted as a mechanism to analyze data for single-subject designs [32]. The literature supports visual inspection as the preferred method of analysis among single-subject designs because it is sensitive and able to capture intervention effects significant to clinicians working outside research labs within clients' natural or typical context [32]. Moreover, the visual analysis approach is preferred because it has lower error rates and is conservative enough to identify reliable treatment effects [32].

In addition to visual analysis, this study used the percentage of non-overlapping data (PND) [33] as an additional analysis tool. PND is a statistical method widely used in behavioral science research, particularly for analyzing the small data sets, which are commonplace with single-subject design studies. PND is calculated by identifying the most extreme data point in the baseline phase (either the highest or lowest value depending on whether the intervention is intended to reduce or increase a behavior). The PND is the percentage of data in the intervention phase, which falls above or below this point based on its intended outcome.

3. Results

3.1. Visual Analysis

The initial step for data analysis for this study was a visual analysis of the data plotted as a figure composed of the scores/ratings from the outcome measures (Daily Caregiver Survey and the Sense Sleep App). The data were evaluated observing changes in level, slope, and variability in data points across each phase for both participants' subjective and objective measures. Figures 1–6 represent the caregiver survey (sleep onset latency, sleep duration, number of night wakings, and morning mood) and the data from the Sleep sense app (sleep score, sleep duration, and deep sleep).

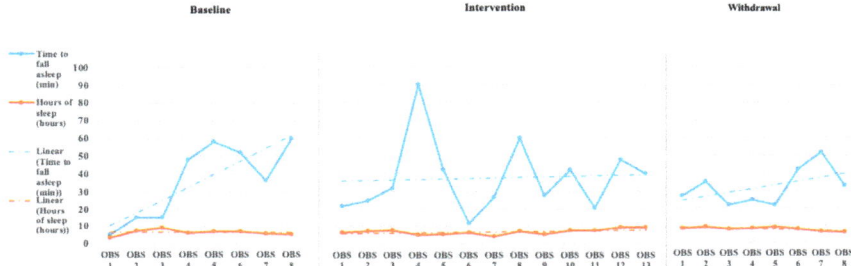

Figure 1. John's caregiver reported sleep onset latency and sleep duration [reported sleep onset latency is measured 0–60 min and sleep duration is measured 0–10 h (OBS = Observation)].

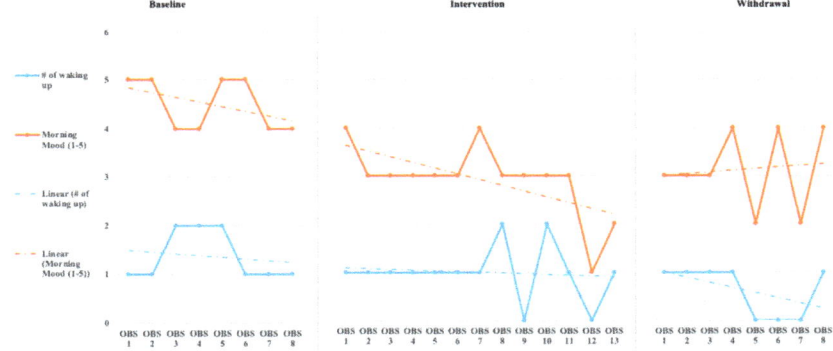

Figure 2. John's caregiver reported number of wakings and morning mood [reported number of wakings is measured 1–5 times and morning mood ratings are 1–5(OBS = Observation)].

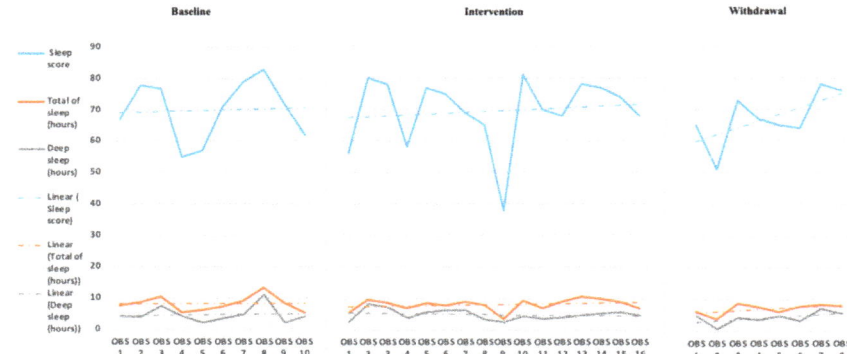

Figure 3. John's Sleep Sense sleep score sleep duration and deep sleep duration [sleep score is measured between 1 and 10, total sleep hours are measured in 0–12 h, and deep sleep is measured in 0–8 h (OBS = Observation)].

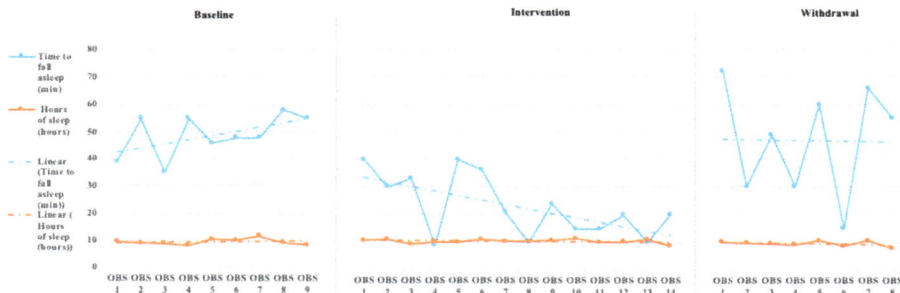

Figure 4. Katie's caregiver reported sleep onset latency and sleep duration [reported sleep onset latency is measured in minutes and sleep duration is measured in hours (OBS = Observation)].

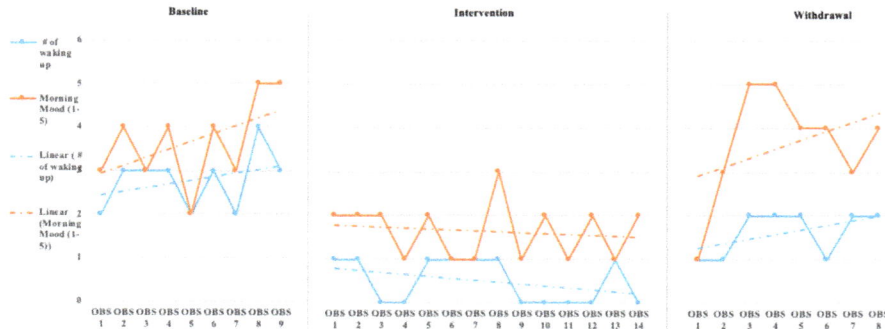

Figure 5. Katie's caregiver reported number of wakings and morning mood [reported number of wakings is measured 1–5 times and morning mood ratings are 1–5 (OBS = Observation)].

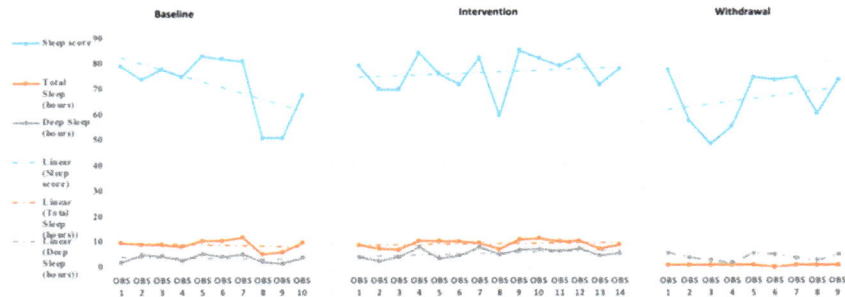

Figure 6. Katie's Sleep Sense sleep score sleep duration and deep sleep duration (sleep score is measured between 1 and 10, total sleep hours are measured in 0–12 h, and deep sleep is measured in 0–8 h).

John's caregiver reported a time to fall asleep during the baseline phase but was reduced to just below 40 min during the intervention and withdrawal phases (see Figure 1). The caregiver's perception of John's total hours of sleep did not see a significant change in level or slope across the phases of the study (see Figure 1). The number of night waking times reported by the demonstrated a downward trend across the baseline and intervention phases and leveled off during the withdrawal phases (see Figure 2). Finally, the caregiver's perception of John's morning mood began relatively level across the baseline and intervention phases but became improved towards the end of the intervention and withdrawal phases (see Figure 2). Visual analysis of the Sleep sense app for John yielded limited changes in slope, level, or variability (see Figure 3).

Analysis of Katie's data through visual analysis yielded notable changes in the caregiver's reporting of time to fall asleep (see Figure 4) during the intervention phase and return to higher levels of approximately 50 min in the withdrawal phase. John's caregiver noted no significant changes in the total hours of John's sleep across all phases. Katie's caregiver reported a slight increase over the baseline phase in the number of night wakings but a small drop and between 1 and 2 times across the intervention phase, returning to higher levels during the withdrawal phase (see Figure 5). Evaluating Katie's caregiver's perception of Katie's morning mood saw a trend on poorer ratings during the baseline phase with a significant improvement in morning mood ratings during the intervention phase with a return to poorer behavioral ratings during the withdrawal phase. Visual analysis of the Sleep sense app for Katie also yielded little changes in slope, level, and variability (see Figure 6).

3.2. Quantitative Analysis

The percentage of non-overlapping data (PND) statistic was calculated to assess treatment effectiveness. Calculations were conducted using Microsoft Excel. Scruggs and Mastropieri [33] provide evaluative criteria for implementing this frequently used analysis method for single-case research. The index of treatment effectiveness is based on the percentage of non-overlapping data using the following criteria: PND ≥ 90% = Very Effective, PND 70–90% = Effective, PND 50–70% = Questionable effectiveness, and PND < 50% = Ineffective. When applying these methods in the current study, the only factor categorized as Effective was for John the morning mood category for Katie the categories time to fall asleep, and the number of night wakings (see Tables 1 and 2).

Table 1. John and Katie percentage of non-overlapping data (PND) analysis of daily caregiver survey.

Daily Caregiver Survey			
A1 Phase—Baseline	PND Baseline—Low	PND Baseline—High	PND Selected
John time to fall asleep (min)	6	60	Low
John Sleep Duration	3.5	9.2	High
John Number of Night Wakings	1	2	Low
John Morning Mood	4	5	Low
Katie Time to Fall Asleep (min)	35	55	Low
Katie Sleep Duration	8.5	11.8	High
Katie Number of Night Wakings	2	4	Low
Katie Morning Mood	2	5	Low
B Phase—Intervention	Number of days PND	PND% out of 14 or 7 days	PND Interpretation
John time to fall asleep (min)	1	0.07	Ineffective
John Sleep Duration	0	0.00	Ineffective
John Number of Night Wakings	2	0.15	Ineffective
John Morning Mood	11	0.84	Effective
Katie Time to Fall Asleep (min)	11	0.84	Effective
Katie Sleep Duration	0	0.00	Ineffective
Katie Number of Night Wakings	13	1.00	Effective
Katie Morning Mood	6	0.46	Ineffective

PND ≥ 90% = Very Effective, PND 70–90% = Effective, PND 50–70% = Questionable Effectiveness, and PND < 50% = Ineffective.

Table 2. John and Katie PND analysis Sense Sleep App.

Sleep Sense App Analysis			
A1 Phase—Baseline Testing	PND Baseline—Low	PND Baseline—High	PND Selected
John Sleep Score	55	83	High
John Sleep Duration	5.3	11.8	High
John Deep Sleep Duration	2.1	11	High
Katie Sleep Score	51	83	High
Katie Sleep Duration	5.1	11.8	High
Katie Deep Sleep Duration	1.5	5.3	High
B Phase—Intervention	Number of days PND	PND% out of 14 or 7 days	PND Interpretation
John Sleep Score	1	0.06	Ineffective
John Sleep Duration	1	0.06	Ineffective
John Deep Sleep Duration	0	0.00	Ineffective
Katie Sleep Score	1	0.06	Ineffective
Katie Sleep Duration	0	0.00	Ineffective
Katie Deep Sleep Duration	7	0.46	Ineffective

PND ≥ 90% = Very Effective, PND 70–90% = Effective, PND 50–70% = Questionable Effectiveness, and PND < 50% = Ineffective.

4. Discussion

The primary aim of this study was to assess the weighted blanket application during sleep for young children with autism with sleep difficulties and tactile and auditory behavioral manifestations of SOR. Does a weighted blanket impact sleep quality among children with autism, sleep disturbances and sensory over responsivity? The findings from the two participants indicate that a weighted blanket had little influence with improving sleep quality through the objective and subjective measures. The findings are consistent with the findings of Gringras et al. [14], Gee et al. [15], Eron et al. [25], and Gee et al. [16]. The existing literature generally does not support that weighted blankets improve sleep quality in children with autism. Occupational therapy professionals working with children with autism, SOR, and sleep disturbances have other therapeutic resources to support improved sleep quality.

4.1. Limitations

The participants were obtained through convenience sampling methods and were comprised of caregiver–child dyads who volunteered to participate in the study via recruitment brochures. Given that the findings are minor and come from a small sample, a generalization of these results cannot be made.

The application of self-report measurement tools created some challenges. The Daily Caregiver Survey lacked any psychometric analysis; however, a critical component of the current study was to provide caregivers an opportunity to offer sleep quality perceptions and rate their child's mood throughout the study. Though the survey ratings offered a caregiver-friendly approach, there are inconsistencies in how the caregivers evaluated each participant's sleep habits, particularly as the caregivers could not be blinded to the study phases.

Culturally, education and healthcare professionals prescribe weighted blankets and vests at 10% of the child's body weight, though there is no empirical data to support such a practice. For this study, it was difficult to determine if the weight of the blankets used were too light or too heavy.

The Hello Sense Sleep App was a proprietary tool, and, unfortunately, the researchers were not provided with its validity and reliability properties despite multiple requests. The authors did not conduct a thorough reliability study prior to implementing the study. The tracking device was typically attached to the participant's pillow, yet if the participant left his/her bed to co-sleep with their parent, removing or dislodging of the tracking device from the pillow or sheet, a gap in the data collection would be introduced.

This highlights a challenge between finding an objective measure that can track sleep outcomes but not cause additional difficulty in tactile SOR that could be caused by a wearable sleep tracking device. This study should be replicated with different and potentially more reliable wearable sleep tracking devices appropriate for pediatric populations with tactile SOR.

Finally, the study's duration, 30 days with 14 days of intervention, may not have been long enough to measure a functional change. The rate at which the participants habituate to having a new/weighted blanket may have been slower than what the study could have captured.

4.2. Recommendations for Future Research

Future research could employ a mixed-methods approach, exploring objective measures either as repeated measures or pre- and post-outcomes related to sleep quality. These outcomes could be paired with caregiver qualitative journals focused on documenting the child's physical activity during the day, evening rituals related to sleep hygiene, and their child's mood the morning after the use of a weighted blanket. A mixed-methods approach could capture missing data from the parent/caregiver's perspective on sleep quality changes while using a weighted blanket with their child. Further research could explore pairing structured sleep hygiene rituals with the child and their parent/caregiver along with a weighted blanket to explore how changes in habits and routines and a sensory-based intervention influence sleep quality in children. More robust research exploring the effectiveness of weighted blankets on improving sleep quality among children with autism is needed. Specifically, research studies using a control (or waitlist) group, larger sample sizes in both the control and experimental group. Further research studies should employ reliable yet affordable objective sleep-related measurement devices that would support the tactile SOR related challenges among some children with autism.

4.3. Key Points for Clinicians

- Weighted blankets for the use of improved sleep quality for children with autism continues to be experimental.
- Clinical professionals using weighted blankets with children with autism should pay close attention to the underlying factors contributing to the child's sleep disturbances (behavioral, biological, environmental, sensory, culture, etc.).
- Clinical professionals need to establish a sound clinical hypothesis for using a weighted blanket with children with autism; monitoring the response to the intervention over time will help support the plan of care on the functional implications of the intervention.
- Clinical professionals should collaborate with the child with autism, medical doctor, and caregiver to identify the underlying mechanisms. Based upon the findings from this and other studies, the use of a weighted blanket to enhance sleep quality in children should be used judiciously; the evidence from this study and other studies indicate that there are more effective approaches to improving sleep quality in children with autism.

Author Contributions: Conceptualization, B.M.G.; methodology, B.M.G.; validation, B.M.G. & K.L.; formal analysis, B.M.G., K.L., J.S. & T.M.; data curation, B.M.G., K.L., J.S. and T.M.; writing—original draft preparation, B.M.G., K.L., J.S & T.M.; writing—review and editing, B.M.G. & K.L.; supervision, B.M.G.; project administration, B.M.G. All authors have read and agreed to the published version of the manuscript.

Funding: This research received no external funding.

Institutional Review Board Statement: The Human Subjects Committee approved the study at Idaho State University (Pocatello, ID) (on 10 February 2017, IRB-FY2016-170).

Informed Consent Statement: Informed consent was obtained from all subjects involved in the study.

Data Availability Statement: The data presented in this study are available on request from the corresponding author. The data are not publicly available due to being stored for only five years in accordance with human subject approval.

Conflicts of Interest: The authors declare that the research was conducted in the absence of any commercial or financial relationships that could be construed as a potential conflict of interest.

References

1. American Psychiatric Association. *Diagnostic and Statistical Manual of Mental Disorders*, 5th ed.; American Psychiatric Publishing: Washington, DC, USA, 2014.
2. Masi, A.; DeMayo, M.; Glozier, N.; Guastella, A. An overview of autism spectrum disorder, heterogeneity and treatment options. *Neurosci. Bull.* **2017**, *33*, 183–193. [CrossRef] [PubMed]
3. Mannion, A.; Leader, G. An investigation of comorbid psychological disorders, sleep problems, gastrointestinal symptoms and epilepsy in children and adolescents with autism spectrum disorder: A two year follow-up. *Res. Autism Spectr. Disord.* **2016**, *22*, 20–33. [CrossRef]
4. Carmassi, C.; Palagini, L.; Caruso, D.; Masci, I.; Nobili, L.; Vita, A.; Dell'Osso, L. Systematic Review of Sleep Disturbances and Circadian Sleep Desynchronization in Autism Spectrum Disorder: Toward an Integrative Model of a Self-Reinforcing Loop. *Front. Psychiatry* **2019**, *10*. [CrossRef] [PubMed]
5. Humphreys, J.S.; Gringras, P.; Blair, P.S.; Scott, N.; Henderson, J.; Fleming, P.J.; Emond, A.M. Sleep patterns in children with autistic spectrum disorders: A prospective cohort study. *Arch. Dis. Child.* **2013**, *99*, 114–118. [CrossRef] [PubMed]

6. Malow, B.A.; Marzec, M.L.; McGrew, S.G.; Wang, L.; Henderson, L.M.; Stone, W.L. Characterizing Sleep in Children with Autism Spectrum Disorders: A Multidimensional Approach. *Sleep* **2006**, *29*, 1563–1571. [CrossRef]
7. Johnson, K.; Malow, B. Assessment and pharmacologic treatment of sleep disturbance in autism. *Child Adolesc. Psychiatr. Clinics N. Am.* **2008**, *17*, 773–785. [CrossRef]
8. Ismael, N.; Lawson, L.M.; Hartwell, J. Relationship between Sensory Processing and Participation in Daily Occupations for Children With Autism Spectrum Disorder: A Systematic Review of Studies That Used Dunn's Sensory Processing Framework. *Am. J. Occup. Ther.* **2018**, *72*, 1–9. [CrossRef]
9. Reynolds, S.; Lane, S.J.; Thacker, L. Sensory Processing, Physiological Stress, and Sleep Behaviors in Children with and without Autism Spectrum Disorders. *OTJR: Occup. Particip. Heal.* **2011**, *32*, 246–257. [CrossRef]
10. Richdale, A.; Schreck, K. Examining sleep hygiene factors and sleep in young children with and without autism spectrum disorder. *Res. Autism Spectr. Disord.* **2019**, *57*, 154–162. [CrossRef]
11. Kirkpatrick, B.; Louw, J.S.; Leader, G. Efficacy of parent training incorporated in behavioral sleep interventions for children with autism spectrum disorder and/or intellectual disabilities: A systematic review. *Sleep Med.* **2018**, *53*, 141–152. [CrossRef]
12. Bodison, S. A comprehensive framework to embed sensory interventions within occupational therapy practice. *AOTA SIS Quarter. Pract. Connect.* **2018**, *3*, 11–17.
13. Mullen, B.; Champagne, T.; Krishnamurty, S.; Dickson, D.; Gao, R.X. Exploring the Safety and Therapeutic Effects of Deep Pressure Stimulation Using a Weighted Blanket. *Occup. Ther. Ment. Heal.* **2008**, *24*, 65–89. [CrossRef]
14. Gringras, P.; Green, D.; Wright, B.; Rush, C.; Sparrowhawk, M.; Pratt, K.; Allgar, V.; Hooke, N.; Moore, D.; Zaiwalla, Z.; et al. Weighted Blankets and Sleep in Autistic Children–A Randomized Controlled Trial. *Pediatrics* **2014**, *134*, 298–306. [CrossRef] [PubMed]
15. Gee, B.M.; Peterson, T.G.; Buck, A.; Lloyd, K. Improving sleep quality using weighted blankets among young children with an autism spectrum disorder. *Int. J. Ther. Rehabil.* **2016**, *23*, 173–181. [CrossRef]
16. Gee, B.; Scharp, V.; Williams, A. Efficacy of Weighted Blankets with young Children with ASD. *Open J. Occupatio. Ther.* **2020**, in press.
17. Reynolds, S.; Lane, S.J.; Mullen, B. Effects of Deep Pressure Stimulation on Physiological Arousal. *Am. J. Occup. Ther.* **2015**, *69*, 6903350010p1–6903350010p5. [CrossRef]
18. Chen, H.; Yang, H.; Chi, H.; Chen, H. Physiological effects of deep touch pressure on anxiety alleviation: The weighted blanket approach. *J. Med. Biol. Eng.* **2011**, *33*, 463–470. [CrossRef]
19. Foitzik, K.; Brown, T. Relationship Between Sensory Processing and Sleep in Typically Developing Children. *Am. J. Occup. Ther.* **2017**, *72*, 7201195040p1–7201195040p9. [CrossRef]
20. Vriend, J.L.; Davidson, M.F.D.; Corkum, P.V.; Rusak, B.; Chambers, C.T.; McLaughlin, E.N. Manipulating Sleep Duration Alters Emotional Functioning and Cognitive Performance in Children. *J. Pediatr. Psychol.* **2013**, *38*, 1058–1069. [CrossRef]
21. Vasak, M.; Williamson, J.; Garden, J.; Zwicker, J.G. Sensory Processing and Sleep in Typically Developing Infants and Toddlers. *Am. J. Occup. Ther.* **2015**, *69*. [CrossRef] [PubMed]
22. Shochat, T.; Tzischinsky, O.; Engel-Yeger, B. Sensory Hypersensitivity as a Contributing Factor in the Relation Between Sleep and Behavioral Disorders in Normal Schoolchildren. *Behav. Sleep Med.* **2009**, *7*, 53–62. [CrossRef] [PubMed]
23. Miller, L.J.; Coll, J.R.; Schoen, S.A. A randomized controlled pilot study of the effectiveness of occupational therapy for children with sensory modulation disorder. *Am. J. Occup. Ther.* **2007**, *61*, 228–238. [CrossRef] [PubMed]
24. Schaaf, R.; Anzalone, M. Sensory Integration with High-Risk Infants and Young Children. In *Sensory Integration with Diverse Populations*; Roley, S., Blanche, E., Schaaf, R., Eds.; Therapy Skill Builders: Cockburn Central, WA, Australia, 2001; pp. 275–292.
25. Eron, K.; Kohnert, L.; Watters, A.; Logan, C.; Weisner-Rose, M.; Mehler, P.S. Weighted Blanket Use: A Systematic Review. *Am. J. Occup. Ther.* **2020**, *74*. [CrossRef] [PubMed]
26. Portney, L.G.; Watkins, M. *Foundations of Clinical Research: Applications to Practice*; FA Davis Company: Philadelphia, PA, USA, 2015.
27. Parham, L.D.; Ecker, C.; Miller-Kuhaneck, H.; Henry, D.A.; Glennon, T.J. *SPM Sensory Processing Measure*; Western Psychological Services: Vancouver, WA, USA, 2007.

28. Owens, J.A.; Spirito, A.; McGuinn, M. The Children's Sleep Habits Questionnaire (CSHQ): Psychometric Properties of A Survey Instrument for School-Aged Children. *Sleep* **2000**, *23*, 1–9. [CrossRef]
29. Lane, A.M.; Terry, P.C. The Nature of Mood: Development of a Conceptual Model with a Focus on Depression. *J. Appl. Sport Psychol.* **2000**, *12*, 16–33. [CrossRef]
30. Hello Inc. *Sense Sleep Mobile Application*; Hello Inc.: Richmond, VA, USA, 2015.
31. Kennedy, C.H. *Single-Case Designs for Educational Research*; Pearson A & B: Boston, MA, USA, 2007.
32. Brossart, D.F.; Parker, R.I.; Olson, E.A.; Mahadevan, L. The relationship between visual analysis and five statistical analyses in a simple AB single-case research design. *Behav. Modif.* **2006**, *30*, 531–563. [CrossRef]
33. Scruggs, T.E.; Mastropieri, M.A. PND at 25. *Remedial Spéc. Educ.* **2012**, *34*, 9–19. [CrossRef]

Publisher's Note: MDPI stays neutral with regard to jurisdictional claims in published maps and institutional affiliations.

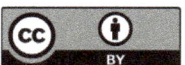

© 2020 by the authors. Licensee MDPI, Basel, Switzerland. This article is an open access article distributed under the terms and conditions of the Creative Commons Attribution (CC BY) license (http://creativecommons.org/licenses/by/4.0/).

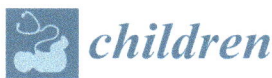

Article

The Utility of Gait Deviation Index (GDI) and Gait Variability Index (GVI) in Detecting Gait Changes in Spastic Hemiplegic Cerebral Palsy Children Using Ankle–Foot Orthoses (AFO)

Majewska Joanna, Szczepanik Magdalena, Bazarnik-Mucha Katarzyna *, Szymczyk Daniel and Lenart-Domka Ewa

Institute of Health Sciences, Medical College, University of Rzeszow, 35-959 Rzeszów, Poland;
joadud@gmail.com (M.J.); szczepanikmp@gmail.com (S.M.); daniel.szymczyk@op.pl (S.D.);
e.domka@op.pl (L.-D.E.)
* Correspondence: k.bazarnik@gmail.com

Received: 27 August 2020; Accepted: 23 September 2020; Published: 25 September 2020

Abstract: Background: Cerebral palsy (CP) children present complex and heterogeneous motor disorders that cause gait deviations. Clinical gait analysis (CGA) is used to identify, understand and support the management of gait deviations in CP. Children with CP often use ankle–foot orthosis (AFO) to facilitate and optimize their walking ability. The aim of this study was to assess whether the gait deviation index (GDI) and the gait variability index (GVI) results can reflect the changes of spatio-temporal and kinematic gait parameters in spastic hemiplegic CP children wearing AFO. Method: The study group consisted of 37 CP children with hemiparesis. All had undergone a comprehensive, instrumented gait analysis while walking, both barefoot and with their AFO, during the same CGA session. Kinematic and spatio-temporal data were collected and GVI and GDI gait indexes were calculated. Results: Significant differences were found between the barefoot condition and the AFO conditions for selected spatio-temporal and kinematic gait parameters. Changes in GVI and GDI were also statistically significant. Conclusions: The use of AFO in hemiplegic CP children caused a statistically significant improvement in spatio-temporal and kinematic gait parameters. It was found that these changes were also reflected by GVI and GDI. These findings might suggest that gait indices, such as GDI and GVI, as clinical outcome measures, may reflect the effects of specific therapeutic interventions in CP children.

Keywords: gait analysis; cerebral palsy; gait variablity index; gait deviation index; ankle–foot orthosis

1. Introduction

Cerebral palsy (CP) with a prevalence of about 2.2/1000 live births is the most common cause of motor disability in childhood [1]. Changes in gait of children with spastic cerebral palsy are often affected by symptoms of spasticity and lower extremity muscle weakness, which limit the patient's ability to walk [2].

The use of ankle–foot orthoses (AFOs) is widely recommended to prevent the development or progression of deformity and to improve dynamic efficiency of the child's gait [3]. There are a wide variety of AFOs used in clinical practice, which are differentiated depending on their design, the material used and the stiffness of that material. Changing any of these three elements will alter the AFO control and this may have influence on the patient's gait [4]. Because of heterogeneity among study designs, AFO types, control conditions, and outcome measures, main effects of AFO on gait of children with CP are unclear. Furthermore, most studies in this area are focused on evaluating a single, specific outcome measure (e.g., step length, ankle range of motion, or knee flexion) rather than the overall effect of AFO use on patient's gait [5].

Three-dimensional gait analysis (3DGA) is commonly used in clinical practice and scientific research for the purpose of objective assessment and description of gait disorders, as well as to plan and evaluate the treatment of children with CP. This method provides a large amount of interdependent data and variables concerning spatio-temporal gait parameters, joint motions (kinematics), as well as joint movement and power (kinetics) in three planes [6]. Given the different gait patterns and pathologies in children with CP, a global analysis is essential in clinical practice. For this purpose, it is useful to summarize and present the results from 3DGA as a single, quantitative, numerical measure that reflects the patient's gait.

One of the models designed to obtain a single measure of the quality of a gait pattern is the gait deviation index (GDI), that measures the subject's gait deviation from a reference, normative data. It is a score derived from 3DGA, which provides a numerical value that expresses overall gait pathology (range 0–100, where 100 and above indicates absence of gait pathology). Every 10-point decrease in the GDI corresponds to one standard deviation from the mean of healthy controls. GDI is calculated based on kinematic parameters [7].

Another gait index, the gait variability index (GVI), is computed based on spatio-temporal parameters. The GVI was intended to be applicable to different patient's groups and diseases severities. It was constructed as a complex measure of nine weighted spatio-temporal gait variables seen in relation to a reference population. GVI value ≥ 100 indicates a similar level of gait variability as the reference population, and each 10-point reduction in the score corresponds to one standard deviation from the reference mean, where lower scores indicate increased gait variability [8,9].

Danino et al. have demonstrated that improvement in temporal and kinematic parameters in spastic diplegic CP children using AFO are not reflected by some gait indices, including GDI [10]. Therefore, the aim of this study was to assess whether the GDI and the GVI reflect changes in temporal and kinematic parameters in spastic hemiplegic CP children wearing AFO.

2. Materials and Methods

2.1. Participants

The study was approved by the Bioethics Committee of the Faculty of Medicine of the University of Rzeszow, Poland (9/2/2017). All children and their parents were informed about the procedures of this study and have signed written informed consent. All measurements were performed in accordance to the Declaration of Helsinki. Participants were recruited from the rehabilitation center for children and youth in Poland. The study population included 37 pediatric patients (19 male and 18 female, with a mean age of 13 years and 7 months). Sixteen children had a right hemiparetic CP and 21 had a left hemiparetic CP (Table 1). All participants walked without additional aids.

Inclusion criteria for hemiplegic CP children were: unilateral, spastic CP as defined by Bax et al. [11]; ability to walk independently at least 10 m; and age between 6 and 18 years. Exclusion criteria were: a previous orthopedic or neurosurgical intervention; botulinum toxin injections within the last 12 months; systemic, anti-spasticity medications; and inability to understand the oral instructions given during the gait analysis. All participants had the posterior leaf spring AFO (PLS) prescribed by their physician. It allows slight plantarflexion, as well as dorsiflexion in stance to promote 'normal' ankle rocker function and to create more dynamic gait. All children had been wearing the PLS for at least 1 month before the gait analysis.

Table 1. Characteristics of the study population

	Number (%)	Mean
Gender		
Male	19 (51.4)	
Female	18 (48.6)	
Age (years)		13.7 ± 4.2
Weight (kg)		47.3 ± 9.1
Height (cm)		155.07 ± 11.5
BMI (kg/m^2)		19.5 ± 2.4
Affected side		
Right	16 (43.2)	
Left	21 (56.7)	
GMFCS I	37 (100)	

BMI—Body Mass Index, GMFCS—Gross Motor Function Classification System.

2.2. Data Collection

3D-gait analysis was performed using a six-camera (120 Hz) movement analysis system with passive markers (BTS Smart, Milan, Italy).

The study procedure included:

- calibration of the system
- anthropometric measurements (body height and weight, lower limbs length, pelvis width and depth of the pelvis, knee joint and the ankle joint width)
- application of the markers according to the modified Davis Protocol
- data recording
- data elaboration and processing using BTS tracker and BTS analyzer software (BTS Bioengineering, Italy).

Reflective markers were placed at defined anatomical points on the pelvis and lower limbs, according to the modified Davis protocol [12]. When walking with the posterior leaf spring AFO and shoes, the lateral malleolus markers were placed on the skin, and the heel and toe markers were placed on the shoes at the positions best projecting the anatomical landmarks (at the level of calcaneous bone tuberosity aligned with the marker at the level of fifth metatarsal). All other markers remained at the same positions throughout the testing procedure. All subjects were asked to walk along a 12-m walkway at self-selected speed, both barefoot and wearing their AFO, in the random order. For each condition, six successive gait trials were recorded and the results of an average of six full gait cycles were subject for further analysis. The same experienced specialist performed these 3DGAs.

Selected spatio-temporal parameters of the gait (the stance phase—percentage of the gait cycle, step length, gait speed, and gait cadence), as well as selected, specific kinematic parameters of the gait (ankle dorsiflexion at initial contact, maximal ankle dorsiflexion at swing, knee flexion at initial contact, maximal knee flexion at swing, knee + hip flexion), for both affected and non-affected lower limb, were computed and analyzed.

2.3. GDI Calculations

The GDI was determined based on the following 9 kinematic parameters: pelvic and hip range of motion in all three planes, knee flexion and extension, ankle dorsiflexion and plantarflexion, and foot progression. GDI values were calculated using the Excel spreadsheet developed by Schwartz and Rozumalski [7].

2.4. GVI Calculations

The GVI was determined based on the following nine spatiotemporal gait parameters: step length (cm), stride length (cm), step time (s), stride time (s), swing time (s), single support time (s), double support time (s), velocity (cm/s), and standard deviations (SDs) of each parameter. GVI values were computed using the Excel spreadsheet developed by Gouelle et al. [9].

2.5. Statistical Analysis

The significance of the differences of the gait parameters in the study group between the two conditions (walking with orthoses and walking barefoot) was calculated using a non-parametric Wilcoxon test. The significance of differences between these two conditions was assessed using a non-parametric, precise version of this test for small samples. The level of significance was assumed at $p < 0.05$. Statistical analyses were performed using Statistica software (StatSoft, ver. 10.0, Krakow, Poland).

3. Results

3.1. Spatio-Temporal Gait Parameters

There were no significant differences between the percentage of the stance phase in the gait cycle (neither for the paretic limb nor for the non-paretic limb), comparing walking with orthoses and without them. On the other hand, statistically significant differences were found in the relative step length for both lower limbs. Significantly worse results are obtained when walking barefoot. Similar relationships were observed in the gait speed. The subjects walked with significantly lower gait speed, when walking barefoot. Additionally, gait cadence in the hemiplegic children group, when using AFO, was significantly reduced ($p = 0.001$) (Table 2).

Table 2. Spatio-temporal gait parameters

Parameters	Mean	SD	p
Stance phase affected leg BF (% of gait cycle)	60.1	3.3	0.127
Stance phase affected leg AFO (% of gait cycle)	59.3	3.3	
Stance phase non-affected leg BF (% of gait cycle)	62.7	4.8	0.764
Stance phase non-affected leg AFO (% of gait cycle)	62.5	4.1	
Step length affected leg BF (cm)	0.60	0.12	0.001
Step length affected leg AFO (cm)	0.66	0.11	
Step length non-affected leg BF (cm)	0.64	0.11	0.002
Step length no -affected leg AFO (cm)	0.69	0.12	
Gait speed BF (m/s)	0.96	0.22	0.002
Gait speed AFO (m/s)	1.11	0.23	
Cadence (step/min) BF	128.7	21.3	0.001
Cadence (step/min) AFO	118.23	21.3	

BF—barefoot, AFO—ankle–foot orthosis, SD- standard deviation, p - significance level

3.2. Kinematic Parameters

Using AFO cause a statistically significant increase in ankle dorsiflexion at initial contact compared to walking barefoot on both, the affected ($p = 0.001$) and non-affected side ($p = 0.019$). Knee flexion at initial contact, when using AFOs, was reduced by 7.6° ($p = 0.038$) on the affected side, while no significant reduction of the knee flexion at initial contact on the non-affected side was observed ($p = 0.09$).

To assess the effect of AFOs on the swing phase, we looked at the maximal ankle dorsiflexion during swing phase and maximal knee flexion in swing phase. Ankle dorsiflexion was significantly increased, when using AFOs, on both sides ($p = 0.002$ and 0.041). Knee flexion was not significantly reduced by the use of AFOs.

To evaluate foot clearance, we calculated the combined maximal flexion of the two joints. Combined flexion at the knee and hip joints showed a significant reduction, for both, the affected and non-affected lower limbs ($p = 0.031$ and 0.046) (Table 3).

Table 3. Kinematic parameters

Parameters	BF Mean	BF SD	AFO Mean	AFO SD	p
Affected leg ankle dorsiflexion at initial contact (°)	−4.73	5.31	4.34	4.26	0.001
Non-affected leg ankle dorsiflexion at initial contact (°)	2.33	5.42	8.27	7.92	0.019
Affected leg max. ankle dorsiflexion at swing (°)	−2.03	7.43	8.29	6.62	0002
Non-affected leg max. ankle dorsiflexion at swing (°)	6.21	7.24	10.32	7.13	0.041
Affected leg knee flexion at initial contact (°)	27.13	9.47	19.48	9.31	0.038
Non-affected leg knee flexion at initial contact (°)	21.42	8.91	17.06	8.67	0.09
Affected leg max. knee flexion at swing (°)	67.04	9.58	64.66	9.41	0.059
Non-affected leg max. knee flexion at swing (°)	65.88	19.58	68.75	7.29	0.106
Affected leg knee + hip flexion (°)	121.21	11.1	114.37	10.82	0.031
Non-affected leg knee + hip flexion (°)	117.19	12.71	112.02	9.23	0.046

BF—barefoot, AF—ankle–foot orthosis.

3.3. Gait Deviation Index

When using AFO, the GDI values increased from 68.6 to 75.1 ($p = 0.029$) in the affected lower limb and from 77.9 to 82.3 ($p = 0.047$) in the non-affected lower limb, which was a statistically significant improvement (Table 4).

Table 4. Changes in GDI

	Mean	SD	p-Value
GDI affected leg BF	68.6	12.3	0.029
GDI affected leg AFO	75.1	10.7	
GDI non-affected leg BF	77.9	10.4	0.047
GDI non-affected leg AFO	82.3	9.7	

BF—barefoot, AFO—ankle–foot orthosis, GDI—gait deviation index.

3.4. Gait Variability Index

The GVI values also increased from 74.2 to 83.1 ($p < 0.001$) and from 78.6 to 86.5 ($p < 0.001$) in the affected and non-affected lower limbs, respectively, which was a statistically significant improvement (Table 5).

Table 5. Changes in GVI

	Mean	SD	p-Value
GVI affected leg BF	74.2	9.48	<0.001
GVI affected leg AFO	83.1	8.74	
GVI non-affected leg BF	78.6	7.67	<0.001
GVI non-affected leg AFO	86.5	8.32	

BF—barefoot, AFO—ankle–foot orthosis, GVI—gait variability index.

4. Discussion

Gait impairments are common in children and adolescents with CP. In spastic hemiplegic CP, decreased walking speed, increased stance phase on non-affected leg, as well as longer gait stride are observed. The stride is usually shorter on affected leg and cadence is increased to maintain gait speed [13]. Gait pattern can be impaired due to motor coordination, balance, and stability problems during walking. Additionally, there are significant differences in kinematic parameters of the hip, knee, and ankle joints, compared to healthy children [14]. For the purpose of the improvement of the dynamic gait efficiency, different types of AFO are recommended for patients with spastic hemiplegic CP [15].

Step length and gait speed are commonly used to assess patient's gait quality [16]. Hayek et al. [17] compared gait of the children with CP, while walking barefoot and with AFOs. In hemiplegic group, stride length increased by 11.7% with AFOs, in both affected (10.2%) and non-affected (12.4%) lower leg. The gait cadence decreased by 9.7%, but walking speed was not improved. Additionally, the authors of this study assessed the impact of using AFOs on the kinematic gait parameters. The ankle dorsiflexion at initial contact increased by 9.4° on the affected side and by 5.87° on the non-affected side, on average. The ankle dorsiflexion at swing was improved about 9.9°, while the knee flexion at initial contact on the affected side was decreased by 8.5° [17]. In their study, Wren et al. compared the gait of children with CP (five patients with spastic diplegia and five with spastic hemiplegia), while walking barefoot and with two types of orthotic devices (dynamic ankle–foot orthosis—DAFO and adjustable dynamic response—ADR AFO). In both types of orthoses children improved stride length, hip extension, and dorsiflexion in swing phase. Using of ADR-AFOs produced better push-off power and knee extension, but the level of activity and patient's satisfaction were higher for DAFOs [18]. Liu et al. evaluated the changes of foot and ankle motion in long follow-up studies (18 months) in the group of 23 children with spastic CP (7 hemiplegic, 16 diplegic), during which patients were using solid ankle–foot orthoses (SAFOs), hinged ankle–foot orthoses (HAFOs), or supramalleolar orthoses (SMO). They observed that the long term use of AFOs can lead to maintaining or improving foot and ankle motion and function [15]. In our study, the step length was longer while the subjects were walking with AFO, comparing to walking barefoot, the gait speed has also improved significantly and the gait cadence was reduced. We have also observed improvement of kinematic parameters, including an increase of the ankle dorsiflexion in stance and in swing phase in both legs. Moreover, the knee flexion at the initial contact decreased significantly only in the affected leg. We did not observe significant changes at the knee flexion during the swing phase, but, both hip and knee flexion range of motion were improved.

In our study, we also evaluated whether the GDI and the GVI can reflect changes in spatio-temporal and kinematic parameters in spastic hemiplegic CP children wearing AFO. GDI and GVI indexes were developed to present how far an individual's gait differs from a normal gait pattern [7,9]. The GDI has been used to assess the gait of children with CP [5,10,16,19,20]. However, we did not find any scientific researches concerning using GVI in this group of patients. This fact encouraged us to check if GVI will be useful to assess changes in the gait of children with hemiplegic CP.

In our study, as it was expected, the value of both gait indices increased, along with the improvement of the selected spatio-temporal and kinematic gait parameters, when the children were wearing AFO. Bickley et al. evaluated two outcome measures: technical surgical goals system (TAG) and GDI and how they reflect changes in postoperative status in children with spastic CP. The TAGs goals have been developed at Shriners Hospital for Children in Huston in 1994 to reflect expected clinical examination and kinematic changes after the surgical treatment. In their study, they observed that using both GDI and TAGs system can improve postoperative assessment in patients with CP at different level of Gross Motor Function Classification System (GMFCS) (I–III). They did not observe any significant differences concerning changes of the GDI results after surgical treatment between different levels (I–III) of GMFCS [19]. Reis et al. showed, that wearing of AFO significantly improves step length, gait speed, and GDI in children with diplegic CP, but only changes in step length was clinically important [16]. A few studies show correlation between GDI and GMFCS. Malt et al. concluded that GDI can be useful to evaluate and present walking impairments in children with spastic CP [6]. Molloy et al. suggest that gait problems may be not well enough recognized when only GMFCS is used; while GDI, as a specific tool for gait assessment, can better reflect functional gait aspects and components [20].

On the other hand, Massaad et al. pointed out that the main clinical utility of GDI is the assessment of the global changes in patient's gait after the intervention, expressed as a single, numerical value, but without specific information about the source or nature of these observed changes [5]. Additionally, Domino et al. showed that the improvement in spatio-temporal and kinematic parameters of gait in children with diplegic CP did not correspond with changes in GDI, Gillette gait index (GGI), or gait profile score (GPS) [10]. In contrast to our study, which has shown that the changes in spatio-temporal parameters and gait kinematics were reflected in GDI and GVI results changes. Galli et al. evaluated the gait of hemiplegic and diplegic children with CP using other gait indices: GPS and gait variable score (GVS), which are also based on kinematic gait parameters. The children were assessed barefoot and while wearing AFO. They concluded that the gait indexes can be useful in evaluation of immediate effects of using the AFOs in hemiplegic and diplegic CP patients, but it was observed only in some GVS parameters—pelvic tilt and ankle dorsiflexion—but not in GPS [21].

The GVI, based on nine spatiotemporal gait parameters was developed and by Gouelle et al. in 31 patients with Friedreich's Ataxia. They showed significant decrease of GVI in patients with Friedreich's Ataxia (70.4 ± 7.9) compared to the healthy subjects (100.3 ± 8.6) [9]. Guzik et al. used GVI for the gait assessment in patients after ischemic stroke. In the control group of the healthy-matched subjects, the GVI scores were 98.34 ± 6.83 for the right lower limb and 96.3 ± 7.19 for the left lower limb and there were significantly different, comparing to the patients after stroke (76.32 ± 7.98 affected leg, 80.74 ± 4.68 non-affected leg) [22]. In the validation study of GVI in patients after stroke in a chronic stage of recovery, the same authors showed that the GVI for the affected and unaffected leg were significantly correlated with the results of clinical functional assessment [23]. Balasubramanian et al. evaluated changes in spatio-temporal gait parameters in two groups of old people, younger and older adults (age < 65 and age ≥ 65, respectively) with GVI. They observed significantly reduced GVI in older adults (91.92 ± 8.75) compared to the younger adults (100.79 ± 7.99). Additionally, they pointed out that low level of functional mobility was correlated with lower value of GVI [24]. GVI score was also validated for patients with mild to moderate Parkinson's disease. The results showed that a mean, overall value of GVI was 97.5 ± 11.7 and mean GVI value for the more affected side was 94.5 ± 10.6 [8]. In our study GVI value while walking barefoot was 74.2 ± 9.48 for affected leg and 78.6 ± 7.67 for non-affected leg and increased significantly when the subjects were wearing AFO (83.1 ± 8.74 for affected leg, 86.5 ± 8.32 for non-affected leg).

Study Limitation

One of the major limitations is the fact that only children at GMFCS level I were included in our study group. Further studies will be necessary, including patients other than GMFCS level I, as well as investigating relationships between the GMFCS level of the children and the quantitative gait assessment, including various gait indices and gait symmetry indices.

5. Conclusions

The improvement of the selected spatio-temporal and kinematic gait parameters, when using AFO, is also reflected in the results of GDI and GVI. These gait indices, being the single, numerical parameter, reflecting changes in gait pattern after various therapeutical interventions, would be also valuable in the clinical practice in the group of spastic hemiplegic CP children.

Author Contributions: Conceptualization, M.J. and L.-D.E.; Methodology, S.M.; Investigation, B.-M.K. and S.M.; Project administration, B.-M.K.; Resources, B.-M.K.; Writing—original draft, M.J. and S.M.; Writing—review & editing, B.-M.K and S.D.; Supervision, M.J. and S.D. All authors have read and agreed to the published version of the manuscript.

Funding: This research received no external funding.

Conflicts of Interest: The authors declare no conflict of interest. The authors of this manuscript have no financial or personal relationships with other people or organizations that could inappropriately bias this work.

References

1. Wingstrand, M.; Hägglund, G.; Rodby Bousquet, E. Ankle-foot orthoses in children with cerebral palsy: A cross sectional population based study of 2200 children. *BMC Musculoskelet. Disord.* **2014**, *15*, 327. [CrossRef] [PubMed]
2. Kerkum, Y.L.; Brehm, M.A.; van Hutten, K.; van den Noort, J.C.; Harlaar, J.; Becher, J.G.; Buizer, A.I. Acclimatization of the gait pattern to wearing an ankle-foot orthosis in children with spastic cerebral palsy. *Clin. Biomech.* **2015**, *30*, 617–622. [CrossRef] [PubMed]
3. Danino, B.; Erel, S.; Kfir, M.; Khamis, S.; Batt, R.; Hemo, Y.; Wientroub, S.; Hayek, S. Influence of orthosis on the foot progression angle in children with spastic cerebral palsy. *Gait Posture* **2015**, *42*, 518–522. [CrossRef] [PubMed]
4. Eddison, N.; Chockalingam, N. The effect of tuning ankle foot orthoses—Footwear combination on the gait parameters of children with cerebral palsy. *Prosthet. Orthot. Int.* **2013**, *37*, 95–107. [CrossRef]
5. Massaad, A.; Assi, A.; Skalli, W.; Ghanem, I. Repeatability and validation of gait deviation index in children: Typically developing and cerebral palsy. *Gait Posture* **2014**, *39*, 354–358. [CrossRef]
6. Malt, M.A.; Aarli, A.; Bogen, B.; Fevang, J.M. Correlation between the Gait Deviation Index and gross motor function (GMFCS level) in children with cerebral palsy. *J. Child. Orthop.* **2016**, *10*, 261–266. [CrossRef]
7. Schwartz, M.H.; Rozumalski, A. The Gait Deviation Index: A new comprehensive index of gait pathology. *Gait Posture* **2008**, *28*, 351–357. [CrossRef]
8. Rennie, L.; Dietrichs, E.; Moe-Nilssen, R.; Opheim, A.; Franzén, E. The validity of the gait variability index for individuals with mild to moderate Parkinson's disease. *Gait Posture* **2017**, *54*, 311–317. [CrossRef]
9. Gouelle, A.; Mégrot, F.; Presedo, A.; Husson, I.; Yelnik, A.; Penneçot, G.F. The gait variability index: A new way to quantify fluctuation magnitude of spatiotemporal parameters during gait. *Gait Posture* **2013**, *38*, 461–465. [CrossRef]
10. Danino, B.; Erel, S.; Kfir, M.; Khamis, S.; Batt, R.; Hemo, Y.; Wientroub, S.; Hayek, S. Are gait indices sensitive enough to reflect the effect of ankle foot orthosis on gait impairment in cerebral palsy diplegic patients? *J. Pediatr. Orthop.* **2016**, *36*, 294–298. [CrossRef]
11. Bax, M.; Goldstein, M.; Rosenbaum, P.; Leviton, A.; Paneth, N.; Dan, B.; Jacobson, B.; Damiano, D. Proposed definition and classification of cerebral palsy. *Dev. Med. Child. Neurol.* **2005**, *47*, 571–576. [CrossRef] [PubMed]
12. Davis, R.B.; Ounpuu, S.; Tyburski, D.; Gage, J.R. A gait analysis data collection and reduction technique. *Hum. Mov. Sci.* **1991**, *10*, 575–587. [CrossRef]
13. Wang, X.; Wang, Y. Gait analysis of children with spastic hemiplegic cerebral palsy. *Neural Regen. Res.* **2012**, *7*, 1578–1584.
14. Guzik, A.; Dużbicki, M.; Kwolek, A.; Przysada, G.; Bazarnik-Mucha, K.; Szczepanik, M.; Wolan-Nieroda, A.; Sobolewski, M. The paediatric version of Wisconsin gait scale, adaptation for children with hemiplegic cerebral palsy: A prospective observational study. *BMC Pediatr.* **2018**, *18*, 301. [CrossRef] [PubMed]
15. Liu, X.-C.; Embrey, D.; Tassone, C.; Zvara, K.; Brandsm, B.; Lyon, R.; Goodfriend, K.; Tarima, S.; Thometz, J. Long-term effects of orthoses use on the changes of foot and ankle joint motions of children with spastic cerebral palsy. *PM&R* **2018**, *10*, 269–275.
16. Ries, A.J.; Novachek, T.F.; Schwartz, M.H. The Efficacy of ankle-foot orthoses on improving the gait of children with diplegic cerebral palsy: A multiple outcome analysis. *PM&R* **2015**, *7*, 922–929.
17. Hayek, S.; Hemo, Y.; Chamis, S.; Bat, R.; Segev, E.; Wientroub, S.; Yzhar, Z. The effect of community-prescribed ankle-foot orthoses on gait parameters in children with spastic cerebral palsy. *J. Child. Orthop.* **2007**, *1*, 325–332. [CrossRef]
18. Wren, T.A.; Dryden, J.W.; Mueske, N.; Dennis, S.W.; Healy, B.S.; Rethlefsen, S.A. Comparison of 2 orthotic approaches in children with cerebral palsy. *Pediatr Phys. Ther.* **2015**, *27*, 218–226. [CrossRef]

19. Bickley, C.; Linton, J.; Scarborough, N.; Sullivan, E.; Mitchell, K.; Barnes, D. Correlation of technical surgical goals to the GDI and investigation of post-operative GDI change in children with cerebral palsy. *Gait Posture* **2017**, *55*, 121–125. [CrossRef]
20. Molloy, M.; McDowell, B.C.; Kerr, C.; Cosgrove, A.P. Further evidence of validity of the gait deviation index. *Gait Posture* **2010**, *31*, 479–482. [CrossRef]
21. Galli, M.; Cimolin, V.; Rigoldi, C. Quantitative evaluation of the effects of ankle foot orthosis on gait in children with cerebral palsy using the gait profile score and gait variable scores. *J. Dev. Phys. Disabil.* **2016**, *28*, 367–379. [CrossRef]
22. Guzik, A.; Drużbicki, M.; Przysada, G.; Szczepanik, M.; Bazarnik-Mucha, K.; Kwolek, A. The use of the gait variability index for the evaluation of individuals after a stroke. *Acta Bioeng. Biomech.* **2018**, *20*, 171–177. [PubMed]
23. Guzik, A.; Drużbicki, M.; Przysada, G.; Wolan-Nieroda, A.; Szczepanik, M.; Bazarnik-Mucha, K.; Kwolek, A. Validity of the gait variability index for individuals after a stroke in a chronic stage of recovery. *Gait Posture* **2019**, *68*, 63–67. [CrossRef] [PubMed]
24. Balasubramanian, C.K.; Clark, D.J.; Gouelle, A. Validity of the gait variability index in older adults: Effect of aging and mobility impairments. *Gait Posture* **2015**, *41*, 941–946. [CrossRef] [PubMed]

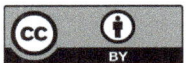

© 2020 by the authors. Licensee MDPI, Basel, Switzerland. This article is an open access article distributed under the terms and conditions of the Creative Commons Attribution (CC BY) license (http://creativecommons.org/licenses/by/4.0/).

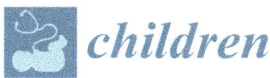

Article

Changes in Ankle Range of Motion, Gait Function and Standing Balance in Children with Bilateral Spastic Cerebral Palsy after Ankle Mobilization by Manual Therapy

Pong Sub Youn [1], Kyun Hee Cho [2] and Shin Jun Park [3],*

[1] Department of Physical Therapy, Kyungbok University, Namyangju-si 425, Korea; psyoun@kbu.ac.kr
[2] AVENS Hospital, Dongan-gu, Anyang-si 307, Korea; 201876402@yiu.ac.kr
[3] Department of Physical Therapy, Gangdong University, Daehak-gil 278, Korea
* Correspondence: 3178310@naver.com; Tel.: +82-43-879-1765; Fax: +82-50-7711-8763

Received: 13 August 2020; Accepted: 15 September 2020; Published: 18 September 2020

Abstract: The aim of this study was to investigate the effect of ankle joint mobilization in children with cerebral palsy (CP) to ankle range of motion (ROM), gait, and standing balance. We recruited 32 children (spastic diplegia) diagnosed with CP and categorized them in two groups: the ankle joint mobilization (n = 16) group and sham joint mobilization (n = 16) group. Thus, following a six-week ankle joint mobilization, we examined measures such as passive ROM in ankle dorsiflexion in the sitting and supine position, center of pressure (COP) displacements (sway length, area) with eyes open (EO) and closed (EC), and a gait function test (timed up and go test (TUG) and 10-m walk test). The dorsiflexion ROM, TUG, and 10-m walk test significantly increased in the mobilization group compared to the control group. Ankle joint mobilization can be regarded as a promising method to increase dorsiflexion and improve gait in CP-suffering children.

Keywords: ankle joint; cerebral palsy; COP; gait; join mobilization

1. Introduction

Cerebral palsy (CP) is a non-progressive upper motor neuron lesion where common motor disability occurs. Other manifestations of CP, such as loss of posture control and lack of movement, may also result in the development of musculoskeletal problem [1,2]. These problems arise because of spasticity and occurs in the hip, knee, and ankle joints [3]. Spasticity is a form of velocity-dependent resistance, or a motor disorder [4]. Children with spastic diplegic CP had greater spasticity at the ankles (more distal part) compared with the knees [5]. The ankle spasticity is related to the limited ankle joint movement [6]. In particular, the limited ankle joint movement in children with CP are closely related to gait and balance performance [7,8]. Therefore, the improvement of balance and gait ability regarding ankle function is one of the goals in rehabilitation for the musculoskeletal problems of children with CP [9,10].

Children with CP are observed to have a limited ankle ROM than typically developing children [11]. The limited ankle ROM of children with CP is also associated with higher tissue stiffness, increased reflexive torque of the gastrocnemius and soleus [11], and spasticity and weakness of the ankle joint [12]. The limited dorsiflexion ROM causes changes in contractile tissue as well as non-contractile tissue and is a common problem for children with CP [13,14].

A limited ankle ROM during gait and balance performance is an identified problem in children with CP [8,15,16]. On the other hand, an ankle ROM improvement may facilitate gait and balance performance [17,18]. For the optimal state of ankle dorsiflexion, it is essential to have a better understanding of the mechanism of limited ankle ROM, and to increase ankle ROM, not only osteokinematics but also arthrokinematics are required. Osteokinematics are simply movements of bones at the joints (flexion/extension, abduction/adduction, and internal rotation/external rotation), and arthrokinematics are small movements of bones at the joint surface (rolls, glides/slides, and spins).

Manual mobilization serves as an important component of neurorehabilitation to treat spasticity and limited ankle movements [19–22]. Manual mobilization is a passive movement performed to relieve pain, complete joint motion, and restore arthrokinematics rather than osteokinematics. Ankle joint mobilization can improve the associated limited ankle ROM characteristic of this condition, especially dorsiflexion [23,24]. Increased dorsi flexion ROM through joint mobilization improved the ankle kinematic changes during walking and [18] and static postural control [25]. These results seem to have a favorable effect on the sensorimotor function and arthrokinematic motion of the ankle [24,25].

Joint mobilization provides a well-suited intervention for ankle rehabilitation, but the effectiveness of a randomized control trial study in children with CP has not been confirmed. As part of manual therapy, there are spine manipulation studies for cerebral palsy [26,27]. Manipulation is a high-velocity (thrust) technique, while joint mobilization is a relatively safe technique with low-velocity techniques [28]. Manual therapy has been supported by several researchers that it can be used as a separate intervention method to treat secondary problems of musculoskeletal system in patients with spasticity (CP or stroke) [19–21,26,27,29–33].

Therefore, the purpose of this study is to investigate the effect of ankle joint mobilization to improve ankle ROM, standing balance, and gait in children with CP.

2. Materials and Methods

2.1. Study Design

This study was single blind, randomized controlled trial with two groups: a mobilization group (ankle joint mobilization) and control group (sham joint mobilization); individuals were randomly assigned using sequentially numbered, opaque-sealed envelopes. The base-line test was performed after obtaining a written informed consent from participants and their legal representatives. The base-line test is ankle dorsiflexion ROM, COP displacements, and gait function (timed up and go test, 10-m walk test). After the baseline-test, children with CP were randomly divided into 2 groups: the mobilization group (ankle joint mobilization, $n = 16$) and control group (sham joint mobilization, $n = 16$). The allocation ratio of the mobilization group/control group was 1:1. The gross motor skills of children with CP can be categorized into 5 different levels using the gross motor function classification system (GMFCS). Since the GMFCS level can provide a confounding interpretation of the results, this study used a stratified block randomization form of the level of GMFCS (1 or 2) [34]. Children with CP were blinded to their treatment. The examiner was blinded to the group allocation. Only the physiotherapist who performed the joint mobilization knew the group to which the participants belonged to. The end-line test was performed after 6 weeks. This study was performed in accordance with the Declaration of Helsinki and research work was approved by the Institutional Review Board of Yong-in University (2-1040966-AB-N-01-20-1812-HSR-127-10).

2.2. Participants

A total of 32 children with CP were recruited from the Bundang Jesaeng general hospital in Gyeonggi do, Korea, February to May 2019. The inclusion criteria were (1) school-aged cerebral palsy children (8 to 14 years) (Mehraban et al. 2016); (2) a diagnosis of spastic diplegia; (3) gross motor function classification system (GMFCS) level I or II [35]; (4) hypomobility according to a 5-point posterior talar gliding test [36]; (5) ability to walk 10 m or more independently; and (6) children with CP to follow verbal directions. Exclusion criteria were (1) a history of selective dorsal rhizotomy and lower extremity orthopedic surgery; (2) botulinum toxin injections in leg muscles during the preceding year; and (3) visual disorder. The detailed study plan is depicted in Figure 1.

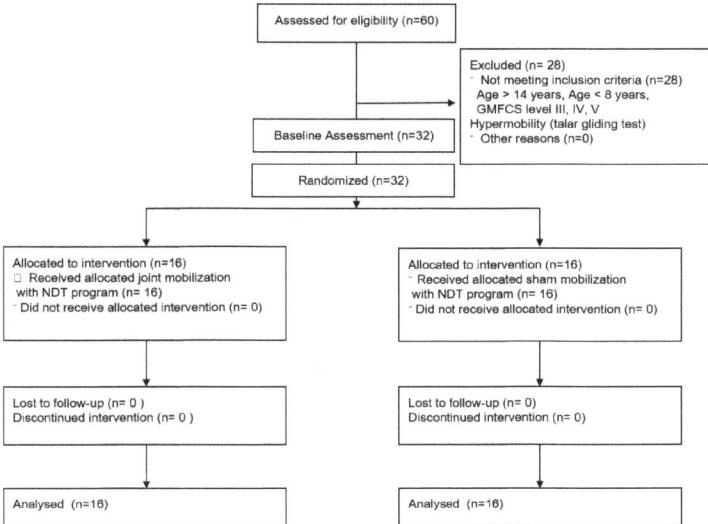

Figure 1. The flowchart of recruitment.

2.3. Sample Size Calculation

G*Power 3.19 (Heinrich Heine University, Dusseldorf, Germany) was used for sample size calculation. The sample size of this study was calculated based on the pilot test. Eight children with CP (four children in the joint mobilization group and four in the sham mobilization group) were involved to calculate the subjects needed for this study. The effect sizes of 1.30 (left) and 1.40 (right) were derived using the mean and standard deviation of dorsi flexion ROM in the supine position among the main outcomes. Based on the effect size of 1.30, input of a confidence level of 95%, and power of 80%, the total required sample size was 22. In this study, 32 participants were selected considering dropout. The initial participants were not included in the sample of 32.

2.4. Intervention Methods

The period of the ankle intervention in this study was 6 weeks. All participants received ankle intervention 30 times (5 sessions per week) over a 6-week period. The mobilization and control groups received the neurodevelopment treatment (NDT) program for 6 successive weeks. The NDT program was performed to improve trunk control. The NDT program consisted of 20 min of trunk muscle exercise and upper extremity exercise (a reaching task of the upper limb for mobility, and trunk control for stability in the sagittal, coronal and transverse planes). The principles of NDT are trunk control in the sitting and standing positions [37]. The mobilization group additionally received (12 min) ankle joint mobilization. The control group additionally received (12 min) sham mobilization.

2.5. Ankle Joint Mobilization

Ankle joint mobilization was performed to improve dorsiflexion ROM. Joint mobilization was performed by one physiotherapist certified in IMTA Maitland concept level 1, with over 10 years of neurodevelopmental treatments experience. After manual evaluation, ankle joint mobilization was carried out in the distal tibiofibular joint, talocrural joint, and subtalar joint. The manual evaluation for ankle joint mobilization procedure is depicted in Figure 2. Manual evaluation to determine the direction of the joint mobilization is as follows. The joint mobilization group recorded the direction of hypomobility among the hypermobility, normal and hypomobility, and performed large-amplitude, rhythmic oscillations (grade III) in the direction of the hypomobility [38]. In this study, except for the distal tibiofibular joint, joint mobilization was applied in the AP direction, and participants received about 50 oscillations per set with 1 min of rest between sets. The rest time was 1 min and applied to both legs for a total of 12 min by applying joint mobilization to the opposite leg during a rest time of 1 min. Therefore, joint mobilization was applied to each of the three ankle joints for 4 min, and the oscillations technique was applied in 2 sets per one leg.

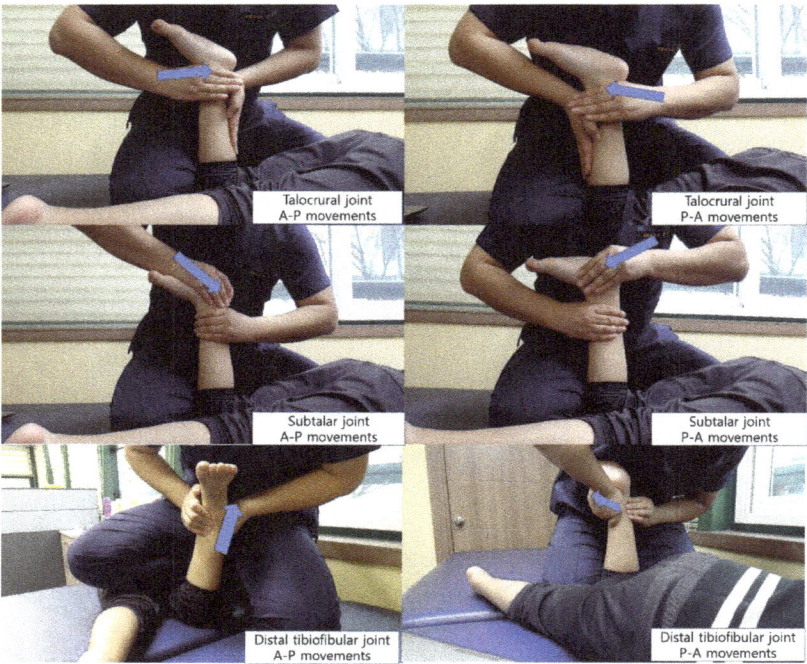

Figure 2. The ankle joint mobilization.

2.6. Sham Mobilization

The sham mobilization visually resembles the joint mobilization. The sham mobilization seems to perform the same action as ankle joint mobilization, but only manual contact is performed because there is no direction of oscillations.

2.7. Assessments

The main outcome measure was ROM in ankle dorsiflexion. The secondary outcome measure was COP displacements and the gait function test. All measurements were performed on the barefoot.

2.8. Ankle Dorsiflexion ROM

Ankle dorsiflexion ROM was measured in the supine position and sitting position [19,39]. For the measurement, a goniometer (goniometer, jamar) was used. To measure the supine position, the participants were in the supine position on a treatment table in a knee extension posture, a sitting position. Measuring of the participants was in the sitting position and with their hip and knees' flexion in 90°. The goniometer axis is located on the lateral malleolus and the stationary arm is located parallel to the fibular head. The movement arm was then the lateral aspect of the fifth metatarsal bone. The examiner fixed the tibial bone and pushed the foot of the participant toward the dorsiflexion.

The dorsiflexion ROM was measured where the end-feel was felt, and no further movement occurred. Measurement of ankle joint ROM using a goniometer has a high reliability [40].

2.9. COP Displacements

COP displacements was measured in a quiet standing position. The COP displacements evaluation is depicted in Figure 3. For the measurement, an AP1153 BioResque (RM Ingenierie, Rodez, France) was used. BioResque is a pressure force platform with 1600 sensors embedded. Participation was achieved by aligning the individuals' bare feet at the 30° leader line indicated above the measurement field of 400 × 400 mm, and holding the standing position for 30 s. At this time, the static sway length (cm) and static sway area (mm^2) of the COP displacement value were measured. COP displacements were measured for an eyes closed and opened condition. The smaller the measured value, the better the standing balance ability.

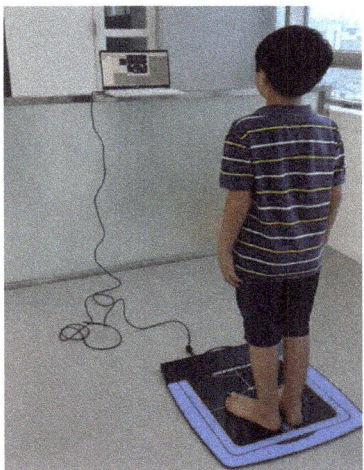

Figure 3. The center of pressure (COP) displacements.

2.10. Gait Function

The timed up and go test was used to assess mobility and balance. The starting position was sitting on a chair without armrests with the hip, knees, and ankle bent in a 90° angle. Participants had to get up from a chair, walk 3 m, return, and sit back in the chair. Measurements were taken after the "start" verbal cue provided by the examiner and recorded until the hips touched the chair. When measuring, the participants were barefoot. The TUG test is suitable for reliable and responsive for measuring functional mobility and dynamic balance of children with CP in GMFCS levels I–III [41]. A 10-m walk test was used to assess gait speed. In this study, a 14-m walkway was used. A stopwatch was used for the measurement, with the starting position in the standing position. When the participant started walking, the time required to walk the 10-m walking distance was measured, excluding the initial point 2 m (acceleration section) and the last point 2 m (deceleration section). The 10-m walk test provides high reliability in children with CP [42,43].

2.11. Statistical Analysis

Data analysis was done using SPSS version 20 software (IBM Corp, Armonk, NY, USA). The confirmation of homogeneity and a normal distribution was verified by means of the K-S tests and independent *t*-tests and chi-square tests. The effects of intervention on dorsiflexion ROM, COP displacements, TUG, and 10-m walk test were examined with a two-way repeated-measures analysis of variance (two-way RM ANOVA). The difference between the initial test and post-hoc test was within-group (time). The mobilization group and control group were between-group (group by time or interaction). If a significant difference appeared in the main effect or interaction, the within-group difference was measured with a paired t-test, whereas a between-group difference was calculated using an independent t-test. The alpha of statistical significance was set at 0.05.

3. Result

The general characteristics confirmed the homogeneity between the two groups (Table 1).

Table 1. General characteristics of the recruited subjects.

Classification	Experimental Group (n = 16)	Control Group (n = 16)	p-Value [b]	p-Value [c]
Gender (male/female)	9/7	10/6	1.000	
GMFCS (Level I/Level II) [d]	6/10	6/10	1.000	
Age (years) [a]	10.81 ± 2.34	11.31 ± 1.78		0.502
Weight (kg) [a]	37.88 ± 8.17	37.13 ± 6.64		0.778
Height (cm) [a]	137.31 ± 9.67	139.06 ± 7.77		0.577

[a] Values are denoted as the mean ± SD. [b] Chi-square test among two intervention groups. [c] Independent t-test among two intervention groups. [d] GMFCS: Gross motor function classification system.

3.1. Change in ROM Dorsiflexion

The experimental groups showed a significant increase in ankle ROM in the sitting and standing position. In addition, the experimental group displayed a significant increase in all ankle ROM compared to the control group (Table 2).

Table 2. Comparison in dorsiflexion ROM pre- and post-test.

Measure/Group	Pre-Test [a]	Post-test [a]	Within-Group Difference [b]	Between-Group Difference [b]
	Lt. Ankle dorsiflexion ROM in sitting position (°)			
Experimental group	14.31 ± 3.00	18.00 ± 2.16	3.69 (2.70, 4.67) *	3.44 (2.42, 4.46) **
Control group	13.63 ± 2.45	13.88 ± 2.83	0.25 (−0.06, 0.56)	
	Rt. Ankle dorsiflexion ROM in sitting position (°)			
Experimental group	14.38 ± 3.16	18.56 ± 2.06	4.19 (2.98, 5.39) *	3.94 (2.71, 5.17) **
Control group	13.69 ± 2.55	14.06 ± 2.77	0.37 (−0.01, 0.76)	
	Lt. Ankle dorsiflexion ROM in supine position (°)			
Experimental group	8.88 ± 2.53	11.56 ± 1.93	2.69 (1.89, 3.48) *	2.31 (1.43, 3.20) **
Control group	7.69 ± 2.50	8.06 ± 2.54	0.38 (−0.10, 0.85)	
	Lt. Ankle dorsiflexion ROM in supine position (°)			
Experimental group	9.00 ± 2.83	12.44 ± 2.50	3.44 (2.50, 4.37) *	2.94 (1.87, 4.01) **
Control group	7.81 ± 2.59	8.31 ± 2.36	0.50 (−0.12, 1.12)	

[a] Values are the means ± SD. [b] Values are the 95% confidence intervals. * Within-group factors: Significant increase compared to the pre-test. ** Between-group factors (Interaction): Significant increase compared to the control group. Experimental group: Ankle joint mobilization. Control group: Sham joint mobilization. ROM: Range of motion.

3.2. Change in COP Displacements, TUG, and 10-m Walk Test

Both the experimental and the control groups displayed a significant decrease in the static sway length and area in the eyes opened condition, eyes closed condition, TUG, and 10-m walk (Table 3). In addition, the experimental group had a significantly increased TUG and 10-m walk test than the control group. However, there was no significant difference between the two groups. However, there was no significant difference between the experimental group and control group in COP displacements (Table 3).

Table 3. Comparison of COP displacements, TUG, and 10-m walk test pre and post-test.

Measure/Group	Pre-Test [a]	Post-test [a]	Within-Group Difference [b]	Between-Group Difference [b]
	Static sway length in the eyes opened condition (cm)			
Experimental group	12.74 ± 2.94	10.23 ± 2.41	−2.50 (−3.32, −1.68) *	−0.79 (−1.85, 0.25)
Control group	12.78 ± 2.77	11.07 ± 2.50	−1.71 (−2.43, −1.86) *	
	Static sway area in the eyes opened condition (mm^2)			
Experimental group	53.35 ± 6.85	36.66 ± 8.73	−16.69 (−21.50, −11.87) *	−2.93 (−9.20, 3.34)
Control group	54.15 ± 7.10	40.39 ± 7.58	−13.76 (−18.19, −9.33) *	
	Static sway length in the eyes closed condition (cm)			
Experimental group	14.28 ± 2.41	11.23 ± 2.37	−3.05 (−4.03, −2.07) *	−0.98 (−2.06, 0.09)
Control group	14.42 ± 2.30	12.36 ± 2.61	−2.06 (−2.61, −1.51) *	
	Static sway area in the eyes closed condition (mm^2)			
Experimental group	59.11 ± 9.14	39.43 ± 9.98	−19.67 (−23.99, −15.35) *	−1.34 (−11.57, 2.89)
Control group	59.83 ± 9.10	44.49 ± 9.84	−15.34 (−21.52, −9.15) *	
	TUG test (sec)			
Experimental group	12.24 ± 2.06	8.50 ± 2.76	−3.74 (−4.45, −3.02) *	−1.95 (−3.12, −0.78) **
Control group	12.78 ± 2.09	11.00 ± 1.68	−1.78 (−2.77, −0.79) *	
	10 MWT (sec)			
Experimental group	10.02 ± 2.26	7.61 ± 1.96	−2.41 (−2.95, −1.86) *	−1.39 (−2.10, −0.68) **
Control group	11.09 ± 1.98	10.08 ± 1.75	−1.01 (−1.51, −0.51) *	

[a] Values are the means ± SD. [b] Values are the 95% confidence intervals. * Within-group factors: Significant decrease than the pre-test. * Within-group factors: Significant decrease compared to the pre-test. ** Between-group factors (Interaction): Significant decrease compared to the control group. Experimental group: Ankle joint mobilization. Control group: Sham joint mobilization. TUG test: Timed up and go test. 10 MWT: 10-m walk test.

4. Discussion

This study found that ankle joint mobilization to improve ankle movements increased ankle ROM and gait function. Moreover, this study demonstrated that ankle joint mobilization is more effective for ankle ROM and gait than sham mobilization. This indicates the importance of ankle joint mobilization in orthopedic management for ankle rehabilitation in children with CP. The strength of this study is that it is the first time in children with CP that joint mobilization was applied to ankle joints in a manual therapy technique. A direct comparison is difficult, but it is consistent with other studies showing that additional joint mobilization is more effective in increasing ankle ROM and gait than conventional rehabilitation [19,24].

When compared with studies regarding the change in passive stretching exercises applied to calf muscles on dorsiflexion ROM [18,44], this study confirmed the positive change effects of passive joint mobilization, such as improved dorsiflexion ROM, TUS, and 10-m walk test. Children with CP exhibit spasticity in calf muscles, so passive stretching has been applied to reduce the spasticity, relaxation, and elongation effect on muscles in previous studies [18,44,45].

However, spasticity exacerbates joint contracture and muscles weakness, as well as changes in the muscle contractile properties [46]. Ankle joint mobilization can be applied to reduce the spasticity of the soleus muscles and [33] restore ankle joint flexibility [19,32]. In addition, ankle joint mobilization causes articular reflexogenic effects, increasing dorsiflexor muscle strength [47]. It has been found that for stroke patients, joint mobilization is a way to increase a variety of ankle ranges of motion rather than stretching exercises [19]. Therefore, joint mobilization can be used as an intervention method to increase ankle mobility in children with CP.

The ankle and knee ROM of children with CP is highly correlated with the energy expenditure index, which means gait efficiency [15]. Ankle joint mobilization increased the ankle dorsiflexion ROM and speed of the sit-to-stand performance [32]. Among the variables measured in this study, the timed up and go test included sit-to-stand. The increased ankle ROM can increase the speed of the sit-to-stand performance, so the timed up and go test may be improved. In addition, ankle joint mobilization with movement can improve gait speed [21]. The posterior talar glide can be increased through joint mobilization [24,48]. Increased posterior talar glide increases dorsiflexion before heel-off and time to heel-off during gait movements [24]. Improving gait velocity through ankle joint mobilization can be considered to affect the dorsiflexion increase during gait movements [19,21,24]. Consequently, ankle joint mobilization improved the gait speed by increasing dorsiflexion during gait movement.

Another finding of this study was that there was no change in the standing balance measurements after additional joint mobilization in children with CP. Ankle joint mobilization can reduce COP displacement by improving sensorimotor function and arthrokinematic restrictions [25]. For the elderly, ankle joint mobilization reduces the surface of standing COP excursions [49]. However, children with CP maintain postural control using a body sway rather than ankle strategy in a quiet standing position [8]. Because of poor postural control, children with CP typically have increased static COP displacement compared to developing children [16]. The wearing of hinged ankle–foot orthoses increased ankle strategy contribution but did not improve postural stability in quiet standing [10]. Therefore, it seems that there was no change in standing balance due to the contribution of body transverse rotation and hip strategies [8,16]. In this study, an NDT program consisted of improving trunk control. An NDT-based trunk protocol is beneficial in improving the trunk control and balance in children with spastic diplegic CP [37]. Therefore, improvement of trunk control by an NDT program decreased COP displacements. Since both groups performed the NDT program, the improvement of trunk control and balance by the NDT program may cause no significant difference between the two groups in COP displacements.

Additionally, the COP displacements in this study evaluated the total COP trajectory. The wearing of hinged ankle–foot orthoses did not change the anterior and posterior displacements but increased the mediolateral displacements [16]. Therefore, to confirm the COP displacements for ankle dorsiflexion ROM increase, it is necessary for future studies to check the mediolateral displacements and anterior–posterior displacements changes, respectively.

Manual therapy applied to growing children can stimulate skeletal growth [30]. Fortunately, no serious or catastrophic adverse events have been reported for children [50,51]. However, due to insufficient evidence so far with regard to manual therapy and adverse events, caution should still be exercised [30,50].

Spine manipulation reduced wrist muscle spasticity in children with CP [27]. Ankle joint mobilization also reduced ankle muscle spasticity in brain injury or incomplete spinal cord injury patients [33]. In this study, ankle joint mobilization, which is safer than spine manipulation, was applied. Joint mobilization can stop the treatments on its own whenever the patient wants to [28]. Therefore, we hope that joint mobilization is often used in clinical settings because ankle joint mobilization is a safe treatment method.

The limitations of this study are as follows. First, our study has a small sample size and it is thus difficult to generalize, and also because our recruitment was limited to GMFCS level I or II. Secondly, our walking speed evaluation method is an evaluation frequently used in clinical settings, but ankle kinematic changes during gait and spatiotemporal analysis (motion capture or inertial measurement units) were not confirmed. To support our hypothesis, we need to further refine and systematically evaluate gait analysis. Finally, this study did not compare long-term effects. Complementing these limitations, future research should investigate the impact of a greater sample size, multiple assessments, and long-term follow-up.

5. Conclusions

The present study shows that additional ankle joint mobilization improves ankle ROM and gait in children with CP. However, the beneficial effect on standing balance was not confirmed. The present study provides new clinical evidence of ankle joint mobilization to increase ankle movements in children with CP. Future research should investigate the impact of a greater sample size, multiple assessments, and long-term follow-up studies.

Author Contributions: Conceptualization, P.S.Y.; Data curation, P.S.Y.; Formal analysis, K.H.C.; Investigation, S.J.P. and K.H.C.; Supervision, S.J.P.; Writing—original draft, S.J.P.; Writing—review & editing, S.J.P. All authors have read and agreed to the published version of the manuscript.

Funding: This research received no external funding.

Conflicts of Interest: The authors declare no conflict of interest.

References

1. Gajdosik, C.G.; Cicirello, N. Secondary conditions of the musculoskeletal system in adolescents and adults with cerebral palsy. *J. Phys. Occup. Ther. Pediatrics* **2002**, *21*, 49–68. [CrossRef]
2. Lomax, M.R.; Shrader, M.W. Orthopedic Conditions in Adults with Cerebral Palsy. *J. Phys. Med. Rehabil. Clin.* **2020**, *31*, 171–183. [CrossRef] [PubMed]
3. Morrell, D.S.; Pearson, J.M.; Sauser, D.D. Progressive bone and joint abnormalities of the spine and lower extremities in cerebral palsy. *J. Radiogr.* **2002**, *22*, 257–268. [CrossRef]
4. Lance, J.W. Pathophysiology of Spasticity and Clinical Experience with Baclofen. In *Spasticity: Disordered Motor Control*; Lance, J.W.F.R., Young, R.R., Koella, W.P., Eds.; Year Book Medical Publishers: Chicago, IL, USA, 1980.
5. Ross, S.A.; Engsberg, J.R. Relation between spasticity and strength in individuals with spastic diplegic cerebral palsy. *J. Dev. Med. Child Neurol.* **2002**, *44*, 148–157. [CrossRef] [PubMed]
6. Hägglund, G.; Wagner, P. Spasticity of the gastrosoleus muscle is related to the development of reduced passive dorsiflexion of the ankle in children with cerebral palsy: A registry analysis of 2796 examinations in 355 children. *J. Acta Orthop.* **2011**, *82*, 744–748. [CrossRef]
7. Rose, S.; DeLuca, P.; Davis, R., III; Ounpuu, S.; Gage, J. Kinematic and kinetic evaluation of the ankle after lengthening of the gastrocnemius fascia in children with cerebral palsy. *J. Pediatric Orthop.* **1993**, *13*, 727–732. [CrossRef]
8. Ferdjallah, M.; Harris, G.F.; Smith, P.; Wertsch, J.J. Analysis of postural control synergies during quiet standing in healthy children and children with cerebral palsy. *J. Clin. Biomech.* **2002**, *17*, 203–210. [CrossRef]
9. Booth, A.T.; Buizer, A.I.; Meyns, P.; Oude Lansink, I.L.; Steenbrink, F.; van der Krogt, M.M. The efficacy of functional gait training in children and young adults with cerebral palsy: A systematic review and meta-analysis. *J. Dev. Med. Child Neurol.* **2018**, *60*, 866–883. [CrossRef]
10. Lintanf, M.; Bourseul, J.S.; Houx, L.; Lempereur, M.; Brochard, S.; Pons, C. Effect of ankle-foot orthoses on gait, balance and gross motor function in children with cerebral palsy: A systematic review and meta-analysis. *J. Clin. Rehabil.* **2018**, *32*, 1175–1188. [CrossRef]
11. De Vlugt, E.; de Groot, J.H.; van der Heijden-Maessen, H.C.; Wielheesen, D.H.; van Wijlen-Hempel, R.M.S.; Arendzen, J.H.; Meskers, C.G. Differentiation between non-neural and neural contributors to ankle joint stiffness in cerebral palsy. *J. Neuroeng. Rehabil.* **2013**, *10*, 1–8.
12. Engsberg, J.R.; Ross, S.A.; Olree, K.S.; Park, T.S. Ankle spasticity and strength in children with spastic diplegic cerebral palsy. *J. Dev. Med. Child Neurol.* **2000**, *42*, 42–47. [CrossRef] [PubMed]
13. Kwon, D.R.; Park, G.Y. Differences in Lateral Ankle Ligaments between Affected and Unaffected Legs in Children with Spastic Hemiplegic Cerebral Palsy. *J. Ultrasound Med.* **2013**, *32*, 313–317. [CrossRef] [PubMed]
14. Huijing, P.A.; Bénard, M.R.; Harlaar, J.; Jaspers, R.T.; Becher, J.G. Movement within foot and ankle joint in children with spastic cerebral palsy: A 3-dimensional ultrasound analysis of medial gastrocnemius length with correction for effects of foot deformation. *BMC Musculoskelet. Disord.* **2013**, *14*, 365. [CrossRef] [PubMed]
15. Ballaz, L.; Plamondon, S.; Lemay, M. Ankle range of motion is key to gait efficiency in adolescents with cerebral palsy. *J. Clin. Biomech.* **2010**, *25*, 944–948. [CrossRef] [PubMed]
16. Rha, D.W.; Kim, D.J.; Park, E.S. Effect of hinged ankle-foot orthoses on standing balance control in children with bilateral spastic cerebral palsy. *J. Yonsei Med. J.* **2010**, *51*, 746–752. [CrossRef]
17. Ahmadizadeh, Z.; Khalili, M.A.; Ghalam, M.S.; Mokhlesin, M. Effect of whole body vibration with stretching exercise on active and passive range of motion in lower extremities in children with cerebral palsy: A randomized clinical trial. *J. Iran. J. Pediatrics* **2019**, *29*. [CrossRef]
18. Wu, Y.N.; Hwang, M.; Ren, Y.; Gaebler-Spira, D.; Zhang, L.Q. Combined passive stretching and active movement rehabilitation of lower-limb impairments in children with cerebral palsy using a portable robot. *J. Neurorehabil. Neural Repair* **2011**, *25*, 378–385. [CrossRef]
19. Cho, K.H.; Park, S.J. Effects of joint mobilization and stretching on the range of motion for ankle joint and spatiotemporal gait variables in stroke patients. *J. Stroke Cerebrovasc. Dis.* **2020**, *29*, 104933. [CrossRef]

20. An, C.M.; Won, J.I. Effects of ankle joint mobilization with movement and weight-bearing exercise on knee strength, ankle range of motion, and gait velocity in patients with stroke: A pilot study. *J. Phys. Ther. Sci.* **2016**, *28*, 689–694. [CrossRef]
21. An, C.M.; Jo, S.O. Effects of talocrural mobilization with movement on ankle strength, mobility, and weight-bearing ability in hemiplegic patients with chronic stroke: A randomized controlled trial. *J. Stroke Cerebrovasc. Dis.* **2017**, *26*, 169–176. [CrossRef]
22. Kim, S.L.; Lee, B.H. The effects of posterior talar glide and dorsiflexion of the ankle plus mobilization with movement on balance and gait function in patient with chronic stroke: A randomized controlled trial. *J. Neurosci. Rural Pract.* **2018**, *9*, 61. [CrossRef] [PubMed]
23. de Souza, M.v.S.; Venturini, C.; Teixeira, L.M.; Chagas, M.H.; de Resende, M.A. Force-displacement relationship during anteroposterior mobilization of the ankle joint. *J. Manip. Physiol. Ther.* **2008**, *31*, 285–292. [CrossRef] [PubMed]
24. Kang, M.H.; Oh, J.S.; Kwon, O.Y.; Weon, J.H.; An, D.H.; Yoo, W.G. Immediate combined effect of gastrocnemius stretching and sustained talocrural joint mobilization in individuals with limited ankle dorsiflexion: A randomized controlled trial. *J. Man. Ther.* **2015**, *20*, 827–834. [CrossRef] [PubMed]
25. Hoch, M.C.; McKeon, P.O. Joint mobilization improves spatiotemporal postural control and range of motion in those with chronic ankle instability. *J. Orthop. Res.* **2011**, *29*, 326–332. [CrossRef]
26. Kachmar, O.; Kushnir, A.; Matiushenko, O.; Hasiuk, M. Influence of Spinal Manipulation on Muscle Spasticity and Manual Dexterity in Participants with Cerebral Palsy: Randomized Controlled Trial. *J. Chiropr. Med.* **2018**, *17*, 141–150. [CrossRef]
27. Kachmar, O.; Voloshyn, T.; Hordiyevych, M. Changes in muscle spasticity in patients with cerebral palsy after spinal manipulation: Case series. *J. Chiropr. Med.* **2016**, *15*, 299–304. [CrossRef]
28. Maitland, G.; Hengeveld, E.; Banks, K.; English, K. *Maitland's Vertebral Manipulation*, 7th ed.; Elsevier: Philadelphia, PA, USA, 2005.
29. Cochrane, C.G. Joint mobilization principles: Considerations for use in the child with central nervous system dysfunction. *J. Phys. Ther.* **1987**, *67*, 1105–1109. [CrossRef]
30. Harris, S.R.; Lundgren, B.D. Joint mobilization for children with central nervous system disorders: Indications and precautions. *J. Phys. Ther.* **1991**, *71*, 890–896. [CrossRef]
31. Brooks, S.C. Role of Mobilization in the Management of Cerebral Palsy. *J. Pediatric Phys. Ther.* **1994**, *6*, 214–217. [CrossRef]
32. Kluding, P.M.; Santos, M. Effects of ankle joint mobilizations in adults poststroke: A pilot study. *J. Arch. Phys. Med. Rehabil.* **2008**, *89*, 449–456. [CrossRef]
33. Pérez Parra, J.E.; Henao Lema, C.P. Effect of joint mobilization on the H Reflex amplitude in people with spasticity. *J. Rev. Cienc. Salud* **2011**, *9*, 125–140.
34. Oeffinger, D.; Gorton, G.; Hassani, S.; Sison-Williamson, M.; Johnson, B.; Whitmer, M.; Romness, M.; Kryscio, D.; Tylkowski, C.; Bagley, A. Variability explained by strength, body composition and gait impairment in activity and participation measures for children with cerebral palsy: A multicentre study. *J. Clin. Rehabil.* **2014**, *28*, 1053–1063. [CrossRef] [PubMed]
35. Palisano, R.; Rosenbaum, P.; Walter, S.; Russell, D.; Wood, E.; Galuppi, B.J.D.M. Development and reliability of a system to classify gross motor function in children with cerebral palsy. *J. Dev. Med. Child Neurol.* **1997**, *39*, 214–223. [CrossRef] [PubMed]
36. Denegar, C.R.; Hertel, J.; Fonseca, J. The effect of lateral ankle sprain on dorsiflexion range of motion, posterior talar glide, and joint laxity. *J. Orthop. Sports Phys. Ther.* **2002**, *32*, 166–173. [CrossRef] [PubMed]
37. Sah, A.K.; Balaji, G.K.; Agrahara, S. Effects of task-oriented activities based on neurodevelopmental therapy principles on trunk control, balance, and gross motor function in children with spastic diplegic cerebral palsy: A single-blinded randomized clinical trial. *J. Pediatric Neurosci.* **2019**, *14*, 120.
38. Maitland, G.; Hengeveld, E.; Banks, K.; English, K. *Maitland's Peripheral Manipulation*; Butterworth-Heinemann: Oxford, UK, 2005.
39. Norkin, C.C.; White, D.J. *Measurement of Joint Motion: A Guide to Goniometry*; FA Davis: Philadelphia, PA, USA, 2016.
40. Elveru, R.A.; Rothstein, J.M.; Lamb, R.L. Goniometric reliability in a clinical setting: Subtalar and ankle joint measurements. *J. Phys. Ther.* **1988**, *68*, 672–677. [CrossRef]

41. Carey, H.; Martin, K.; Combs-Miller, S.; Heathcock, J.C. Reliability and responsiveness of the timed up and go test in children with cerebral palsy. *J. Pediatric Phys. Ther.* **2016**, *28*, 401–408. [CrossRef]
42. Chrysagis, N.; Skordilis, E.K.; Koutsouki, D. Validity and clinical utility of functional assessments in children with cerebral palsy. *J. Arch. Phys. Med. Rehabil.* **2014**, *95*, 369–374. [CrossRef]
43. Bahrami, F.; Dehkordi, S.N.; Dadgoo, M. Inter and intra rater reliability of the 10 meter walk test in the community dweller adults with spastic cerebral palsy. *J. Iran. J. Child Neurol.* **2017**, *11*, 57.
44. Zhao, H.; Wu, Y.N.; Hwang, M.; Ren, Y.; Gao, F.; Gaebler-Spira, D.; Zhang, L.Q. Changes of calf muscle-tendon biomechanical properties induced by passive-stretching and active-movement training in children with cerebral palsy. *J. Appl. Physiol.* **2011**, *111*, 435–442. [CrossRef]
45. Flett, P.; Stern, L.; Waddy, H.; Connell, T.; Seeger, J.; Gibson, S. Botulinum toxin A versus fixed cast stretching for dynamic calf tightness in cerebral palsy. *J. Paediatr. Child Health* **1999**, *35*, 71–77. [CrossRef] [PubMed]
46. Gracies, J.M. Pathophysiology of spastic paresis. I: Paresis and soft tissue changes. *Muscle Nerve* **2005**, *31*, 535–551. [CrossRef] [PubMed]
47. Ersoy, U.; Kocak, U.Z.; Unuvar, E.; Unver, B. The Acute Effect of Talocrural Joint Mobilization on Dorsiflexor Muscle Strength in Healthy Individuals: A Randomized Controlled Single-Blind Study. *J. Sport Rehabil.* **2019**, *28*, 601–605. [CrossRef] [PubMed]
48. Vicenzino, B.; Branjerdporn, M.; Teys, P.; Jordan, K. Initial changes in posterior talar glide and dorsiflexion of the ankle after mobilization with movement in individuals with recurrent ankle sprain. *J. Orthop. Sports Phys. Ther.* **2006**, *36*, 464–471. [CrossRef]
49. Chevutschi, A.; D'houwt, J.; Pardessus, V.; Thevenon, A. Immediate effects of talocrural and subtalar joint mobilization on balance in the elderly. *J. Physiother. Res. Int.* **2015**, *20*, 1–8. [CrossRef]
50. Humphreys, B.K. Possible adverse events in children treated by manual therapy: A review. *J. Chiropr. Osteopathy* **2010**, *18*, 12. [CrossRef]
51. Driehuis, F.; Hoogeboom, T.J.; Nijhuis-van der Sanden, M.W.; de Bie, R.A.; Staal, J.B. Spinal manual therapy in infants, children and adolescents: A systematic review and meta-analysis on treatment indication, technique and outcomes. *PLoS ONE* **2019**, *14*, e0218940. [CrossRef]

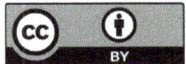

© 2020 by the authors. Licensee MDPI, Basel, Switzerland. This article is an open access article distributed under the terms and conditions of the Creative Commons Attribution (CC BY) license (http://creativecommons.org/licenses/by/4.0/).

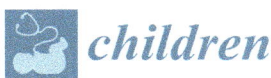

Article

Effect of Functional Progressive Resistance Exercise on Lower Extremity Structure, Muscle Tone, Dynamic Balance and Functional Ability in Children with Spastic Cerebral Palsy

Hye-Jin Cho [1] and Byoung-Hee Lee [2],*

[1] Graduate School of Physical Therapy, Sahmyook University, Seoul 01795, Korea; manje50@hanmail.net
[2] Department of Physical Therapy, Sahmyook University, Seoul 01795, Korea
* Correspondence: 3679@syu.ac.kr; Tel.: +82-(2)-3399-1634

Received: 4 June 2020; Accepted: 28 July 2020; Published: 31 July 2020

Abstract: The purpose of this study was to investigate the effects of functional progressive resistance exercise (FPRE) on muscle tone, dynamic balance and functional ability in children with spastic cerebral palsy. Twenty-five subjects were randomized into two groups: the FPRE group ($n = 13$) and the control group ($n = 12$). The experimental group participated in an FPRE program for 30 min per day, three times per week for six weeks. Knee extensor strength, rehabilitative ultrasound imaging (RUSI), muscle tone, dynamic balance, and functional ability was evaluated. The results showed statistically significant time × group interaction effects on the dominant side for knee extensor strength and cross-sectional area (CSA) in RUSI ($p < 0.05$). On both sides for thickness of the quadriceps (TQ) in RUSI, muscle tone and dynamic balance were statistically significant time × group interaction effects ($p < 0.05$). Additionally, knee extensor strength, CSA, TQ in RUS, muscle tone, dynamic balance and gross motor function measure (GMFM) in functional ability were significantly increased between pre- and post-intervention within the FPRE group ($p < 0.05$). The results suggest that FPRE is both feasible and beneficial for improving muscle tone, dynamic balance and functional ability in children with spastic cerebral palsy.

Keywords: cerebral palsy; functional progressive resistance exercise; muscle strength; muscle tone

1. Introduction

Cerebral palsy has been defined as a nonprogressive disorder that affects the development of movement and posture, causing limitation of activity in the developing fetus or infant. Disturbances of sensation, cognition, communication, perception and behavior by seizure disorder are the most common disorders associated with cerebral palsy (CP) [1]. CP can be classified based on the type of movement disorder as spastic, athetoid, ataxic and mixed; CP can also be classified based on the area of the body involved as hemiplegia, diplegia and quadriplegia [2], in which spastic diplegia is the most common type [3]. Spasticity, caused by damage to the pyramidal parts of the brain, is defined as a velocity-dependent resistance to stretch [2]. Due to spasticity, the onset of postural muscle activity in children with CP is delayed compared to normally developing children. In addition, impairment was observed upon sequencing of multiple muscle; additionally, there is an increased level of co-activation of agonist and antagonist muscles at a joint, which results in reduction of balance [4].

CP is a neurological disorder that can cause secondary changes in the musculoskeletal system, such as decreased muscle strength, tightness or contractures around joints and abnormalities in both bony structures and gait [5]. Therefore, children with CP show weakened muscle due to lack of motor unit activation and thickness in 50% of small muscles, compared to normally developing children. Infants with CP have reduced knee extensor and ankle plantar flexor strength than normally developing infants [6], and CP has reduced rectus femoris thickness compared with normally developing children [7]. The thickness of the quadriceps muscle, indicative of lower extremity strength, has an effect on the quality of life of children with CP; indeed, a study has shown that children with thicker quadricep muscles participated more in community-related activities [8]. Based on this result, lower extremity strengthening should be emphasized in the rehabilitation of children with CP.

Many methods of muscle strengthening are recommended for children with CP, such as functional progressive resistance exercise (FPRE) [9], isokinetic training [10], bicycle and treadmill exercise [11], weight training [12], aquatic training [13], sports and recreation [14] and electrotherapy [15]. Until recently, strength training in children with CP was considered inappropriate, as it was believed to lead to increased spasticity or abnormal movement patterns.

The muscles of children with CP have an increased amount of collagen, which hinders movement. This increase in collagen is responsible for contracture development, thereby affecting the passive viscoelastic features of muscle and exerting an impact on the internal resistance of muscle when passive movement of the joint is performed [16]. A weak agonist muscle may not allow full lengthening of the spastic antagonist muscle, leading to contracture development, and an increase in passive tension leads to muscle weakness [17].

FPRE can improve lower limb muscle strength and improve function in children with CP without increasing spasticity [18]. Essentially, FPRE provides sufficient resistance so that a low number of repetitions (usually 8–12) can be completed before fatigue sets in [19]. FPRE includes exercises, such as sit to stand, half-kneeling standing and side step-up [20]. A study on antigravity close kinematic chain exercise [21] showed that FPRE effectively increases lower muscle strength, thereby facilitating lower extremity co-contraction and allowing agonist and antagonist muscles to work effectively; this leads to reduction of muscle tone in the lower extremity [22].

This study aims to contribute to the improvement of rehabilitation in children with spastic CP by investigating the effect of FPRE on knee extensor strength, myoarchitectonic of the quadriceps, muscle tone, dynamic balance and functional ability of the lower extremity.

2. Materials and Methods

2.1. Methods

The subjects were selected from 28 children with diplegia CP undergoing physical therapy at K Hospital in Gyeonggi-do, Korea. The specific selection criteria of the study subjects were children between the ages of 6 and 13 years diagnosed with diplegic CP, who were able to follow the researcher's instructions and had a GMFCS (gross motor function classification system) level between I and III [23]. Children were excluded if they had unstable seizures, had received treatment for spasticity or any surgical procedure up to 3 months (for botulinum toxin type A injections) to 6 months (for surgery) prior to the start of the study—or if they suffered from other diseases that interfered with physical activity [24].

Subject's age, height, weight, BMI and GMFCS level were measured prior to each intervention to apply the appropriate amount of weight for each intervention. All subjects picked a black or white stone from a box containing 28 stones. Subjects were randomly divided into an experimental group or a control group, with 14 subjects in each group.

One week before training and one week after training proceeded the evaluation. The intervention group performed FPRE for 30 min per day, three times per week, during a period of 6 weeks. For the control group, a conventional physical therapy program was applied instead of FPRE. However, during the intervention, one subject in the FPRE group had to drop out due to their health condition and two subjects in the control group were excluded because they moved out of town.

This study was conducted with the approval of the research institutional review board of Sahmyook University (2-7001793-AB-N-012018014HR) and it was registered (KCT0005055) as a Clinical Research Information Service (CRIS) in Republic of Korea. The objective and the procedures performed in the study were explained to the subjects' parents, and all of the subjects' parents provided informed consent for inclusion in the study. Therefore, this study was conducted according to the ethical principles of the Declaration of Helsinki.

2.2. Experimental Methods

2.2.1. Functional Progressive Resistance Exercise

The FPRE program was modified based on circuit training that follows the program used by US National strength and conditioning association (NSCA). Strength training must be individualized and should involve a progressive increase in intensity to be successful, thereby stimulating strength gains that are greater than those associated with normal growth and development [25]. The FPRE can be used to bear, overcome or resist force, such as body weight, free weights or machines. The exercise was conducted three times per week for 6 weeks. Each exercise was comprised of 5 min of warmup exercise followed by three different types of exercise. Exercise repetition increased to five times in the first two weeks, 10 times in the subsequent 2 weeks and 15 times in the last two weeks. More specifically, according to subject's participation, body weight and exercise repetition will be increased every two weeks by 5%, 10% and 35% based on their body weight. According to each subject's performance both weight and repetition would be increased; however, in the event that the subjects were unable to follow the increase in exercise repetition or weights used during exercise, the level of difficulty would remain the same.

In the following protocol, three circuit exercises were included: sit to stand, half-kneeling standing up and side step-up. In the sit to stand exercise, the child sits on a bench with no back rest. In the starting position, the child's back, knee and ankle need to be flexed at a 90° angle and their ankles should be in contact with the floor. From the starting position, the subject would be instructed by the physical therapist to stand up slowly from the bench. In the half-kneeling standing exercise, the child is sitting in a half-kneeling position without any external support. From this starting position, the child gradually pushes forward to stand up while the weight is shifted forward on the front leg. In the side step-up exercise, the child climbs up a 15 cm staircase sideways [26]. Between each circuit, 30 s to 1 min of rest time was given to subjects. Longer rest times were given to subjects with lower GMFCS scores to reduce stress. A cooling down exercise and range of motion stretching was held in the final 2 min (Table 1).

Table 1. Functional progressive resistance exercise protocol.

FPRE	Exercise Protocol	Duration
Warmup	Range of motion mobilization, stretching	3 min
% weight [a]	Sit to stand	5 min
	Rest	
% weight [a]	Half-kneeling standing up, side-step-up	10 min
	Rest	
Body weight	Half-kneeling standing up, side-step-up	10 min
Cooldown	Range of motion mobilization, stretching	2 min

FPRE—functional progressive resistive exercise; [a] Progressively increased to five times, 5% weight in 1–2 weeks; 10 times, 10% weight in 3–4 weeks; 15 times, 35% weight in 5–6 weeks.

2.2.2. Conventional Therapy

Conventional therapy, which was prescribed by a rehabilitation doctor in K hospital, included FES, standing frame and mat exercise. In the control group, conventional therapy had a duration of 30 min three times per a week for 6 weeks. The instructor for each exercise was a pediatric physiotherapist with 3 or more years of work experience.

2.3. Outcome Measurements

2.3.1. Knee Extensor Strength

In this study, knee extensor strength was measured with a handheld dynamometer FPX 50 (Wagner, Inc., Greenwich, CT, USA, 2017) before and after the intervention by therapists who received 40 min of education regarding proper use of the hand hold dynamometer. The measurement of the knee extensor was performed with the subject in a sitting position, with knee and hip in a 90-degree flexion without back support. Since gravity effects can result in measurement errors, all actions were tested in gravity-neutralized Bryant positions [27]. Subjects were required to place both hands on their lap and HHD was placed 3 cm above the ankle joint. Three attempts were made to find the mean value for the knee extensor strength measurement. The reliability ICC was 0.91 [28].

2.3.2. Rehabilitative Ultrasound Imaging

The use of ultrasound imaging (USI) to aid rehabilitation of neuromusculoskeletal disorders or rehabilitative ultrasound imaging (RUSI), is defined as 'a procedure used by physical therapists to evaluate muscle and related soft tissue morphology and function during exercise and physical tasks [29]. In this study, morphology of the quadriceps muscle was measured with portable ultrasound, Medison Mysono P-US system (U5, Samsung Medison, Seoul, Korea). The cross-sectional area of the rectus femoris and the thickness of the quadriceps, from the top of the rectus femoris to the bottom of the vastus intermedius, were measured three times on both legs. Regarding the reliability of this test, the interrater reliability ICC was 0.87–0.97, while the intra-rater reliability ICC was 0.78–0.95 in younger people [30].

2.3.3. Muscle Tone

In this study, Electronic goniometer, Baseline 12-1027 Absolute+Axis digital goniometer (Baseline, Inc., New York, NY, USA, 2016) was used to measure the popliteal range of motion in passive, speed and active. In supine position ipsilateral hip and knee were flexed to 90° and the knee maximally passively extended to the point of mild resistance, active range of motion and range of motion with velocity were also measured in same positions [31]. To provide consistent rate and provide highly reliable measures, it was calculated as the mean of three trials. The ICC for this test was 0.999 [32].

2.3.4. Dynamic Balance

In this study, dynamic balance was examined using the functional reach test (FRT). The FRT was performed with a leveled yardstick that was mounted on the wall at the height of the patient's acromion level in the unaffected arm while sitting in a chair. Hips, knees and ankles were positioned at a 90-degree flexion, with feet positioned flat on the floor. The initial reach is measured with the patient sitting against the back of the chair with the upper extremity flexed to 90 degrees; the measurement was made from the distal end of the third metacarpal along the yardstick [33]. The FRT measures the maximum distance that subjects can reach forward (F-FRT) and sideways (S-FRT) with their arm while maintaining a fixed base of support in the sitting position. The distance was measured in centimeters to the second digit. The interrater reliability ICC of this test was 0.99 and intra-rater reliability ICC was 0.97 [34].

2.3.5. Functional Ability

Functional ability was scored with the GMFM-88. The gross motor function measure (GMFM) is a five-level classification system that appears to be valid in assessing the child's current motor functions, including laying/rolling, sitting, crawling/kneeling, standing and walking/running/jumping and is thought to have prognostic potential, i.e., early classification of a child could help determine long-term motor function [35]. The reliability ICC ranged from 0.92 to 0.99 for all dimensions and total scores [36].

2.4. Statistical Analysis

All demographic variables of subjects displayed normal distribution. SPSS version 25.0 statistical software (IBM, Chicago, IL, USA) was used for analysis of all statistical values. Results are presented as mean ± standard deviation. The general characteristics of two groups were analyzed using chi-squared analysis and the independent *t*-test. The interaction effect between group and time was assessed using a repeated-measures analysis of variance. A paired *t*-test was used to compare the results before and after the intervention in each FPRE group and control group. For all tests, the level of statistical significance was set to 0.05.

3. Results

3.1. General Characteristics of Subject

Demographic characteristics are shown in Table 2. No significant differences were observed in the baseline value between the FPRE group and control group for all parameters.

Table 2. General Characteristics of subjects ($N = 25$).

Characteristics	FPRE Group ($n = 13$)	CG Group ($n = 12$)	$X^2/t(p)$
Gender (male/female)	4/9	8/4	1.845(0.078)
Dominant/non-dominant	7/6	9/3	1.082(0.290)
Age (years)	5.54 ± 1.808	7.17 ± 2.167	−2.046(0.052)
Height (cm)	108.54 ± 14.65	117.10 ± 12.73	−1.553(0.134)
Weight (kg)	19.56 ± 7.40	24.37 ± 7.73	−1.587(0.126)
BMI (Z-score)	0.14 ± 1.76	0.60 ± 1.01	−0.790(0.406)
GMFCS level	2.08 ± 0.862	2.33 ± 1.073	−0.661(0.515)
GMFM score	69.98 ± 21.55	68.15 ± 27.15	0.187(0.853)

Values expressed as mean ± standard deviation; FPRE—functional progressive resistive exercise; CG—control group; GMFCS—gross motor function classification system; GMFM—gross motor function measure.

3.2. Comparison of Knee Extensor Muscle Strength between the FPRE Group and Control Group

Statistically significant time factor effects on knee extensor muscle strength of the dominant and non-dominant side ($p < 0.05$) were observed, as well statistically significant time × group interaction effects on the knee extensor muscle strength of the dominant side ($p < 0.05$).

A paired *t*-test revealed statistically significant improvements on the knee extensor muscle strength of the dominant and non-dominant side in the FPRE group ($p < 0.05$). However, in the control group, the mean value between the pre and posttest showed no significant difference (Table 3).

Table 3. Knee extensor muscle strength ($N = 25$).

Muscle Strength		FPRE Group ($n = 13$)	CG Group ($n = 12$)	Time F(p)	Group F(p)	Time × Group F(p)
Non-dominant (N)	Pretest	40.62 ± 30.61	34.54 ± 28.55	8.367(0.008)	0.490(0.491)	0.629(0.436)
	Posttest	51.24 ± 33.58	40.59 ± 29.50			
	t(p)	−2.196(0.048)	−2.078(0.062)			
Dominant (N)	Pretest	30.45 ± 27.57	41.61 ± 34.00	8.368(0.008)	0.060(0.808)	5.412(0.029)
	Posttest	52.39 ± 33.13	43.12 ± 32.17			
	t(p)	−3.065(0.010)	−0.590(0.567)			

Values expressed as mean ± standard deviation; FPRE—functional progressive resistance exercise; CG—control group.

3.3. Comparison of the Structure of the Quadriceps between the FPRE Group and the Control Group

Changes in the lower extremity, specifically the quadriceps, were assessed with portable RUSI. Table 4 presents the results observed in the FPRE group and the control group. Statistically significant time factor effects on the mean value of TQ and CSA of the dominant and non-dominant side were observed ($p < 0.05$), as well as statistically significant group factor effects on the CSA of the dominant and non-dominant side. Additionally, statistically significant time × group interaction effects were observed on the mean value of TQ of the dominant and non-dominant side and CSA of the dominant side ($p < 0.05$).

Table 4. Comparison of the structure of the quadriceps between the of functional progressive resistance exercise (FPRE) group and control group ($N = 25$).

	Structure		FPRE Group ($n = 13$)	CG Group ($n = 12$)	Time F(p)	Group F(p)	Time × Group F(p)
TQ	Non-dominant	Pretest Posttest t(p)	1.39 ± 0.27 1.98 ± 0.316 −8.544(0.000)	1.46 ± 0.29 1.66 ± 0.34 −1.610(0.136)	32.191(0.000)	1.427(0.244)	7.834(0.010)
	Dominant	Pretest Posttest t(p)	1.41 ± 0.24 1.95 ± 0.29 −11.284(0.000)	1.40 ± 0.308 1.70 ± 0.35 −4.578(0.001)	109.633(0.000)	1.308(0.265)	8.978(0.006)
CSA	Non-dominant	Pretest Posttest t(p)	3.41 ± 0.807 4.54 ± 0.97 −3.390(0.005)	3.22 ± 0.57 3.49 ± 1.05 −0.987(0.345)	10.288(0.004)	5.240(0.032)	3.830(0.063)
	Dominant	Pretest Posttest t(p)	3.64 ± 0.64 4.63 ± 0.99 −3.110(0.009)	3.29 ± 0.66 3.45 ± 0.89 −0.722(0.485)	8.578(0.008)	8.549(0.008)	4.451(0.044)

Values expressed as mean ± standard deviation; FPRE—functional progressive resistive exercise; CG—control group; TQ—thickness of the quadriceps; CSA—cross-sectional area of the rectus femoris.

A paired *t*-test revealed a statistically significant increase on the mean value of TQ and CSA of the dominant and non-dominant sides in the FPRE group after the intervention ($p < 0.05$). However, the mean value of TQ of the dominant side significantly increased after the intervention in the control group ($p < 0.05$).

3.4. Comparison of Muscle Tone According to Popliteal Angle in Passive, Speed and Active Ranges of Motion between FPRE and Control Group

Popliteal angles in passive, speed and active ranges of motion were assessed to evaluate the effects of FPRE on lower leg range of motion and strength. Statistically significant time factor effects on the PA-P of the dominant side and PA-A of the dominant and non-dominant side were observed ($p < 0.05$). Statistically significant group factor effects were observed on the PA-P of the dominant and non-dominant side, as well as PA-S of the non-dominant side ($p < 0.05$). In addition, statistically significant time × group interaction effects were observed on the PA-P, PA-S and PA-A of the dominant and non-dominant sides ($p < 0.05$).

A paired *t*-test revealed a statistically significant increase after the intervention on the PA-P and PA-A of the dominant and non-dominant sides and PA-S of the non-dominant side in the FPRE group ($p < 0.05$). However, in the control group, the mean value between the pre and posttest showed no significant difference (Table 5).

Table 5. Muscle tone popliteal angle in passive, speed and active ranges of motion ($N = 25$).

Popliteal Angle			FPRE Group ($n = 13$)	CG Group ($n = 12$)	Time F(p)	Group F(p)	Time × Group F(p)
PA-P (degree)	Non-dominant	Pretest	151.17 ± 17.82	142.92 ± 18.07	0.241(0.628)	4.464(0.046)	8.994(0.006)
		Posttest	158.57 ± 14.66	137.61 ± 21.35			
		t(p)	−2.454(0.030)	1.792(0.101)			
	Dominant	Pretest	153.39 ± 15.86	144.68 ± 15.96	4.747(0.040)	6.289(0.020)	4.890(0.037)
		Posttest	163.27 ± 10.19	144.61 ± 16.32			
		t(p)	−2.745(0.018)	0.028(0.978)			
PA-S (degree)	Non-dominant	Pretest	141.32 ± 13.27	136.49 ± 19.11	0.390(0.538)	5.721(0.025)	8.909(0.007)
		Posttest	152.45 ± 13.11	129.21 ± 20.01			
		t(p)	−2.879(0.014)	1.495(0.163)			
	Dominant	Pretest	142.24 ± 15.31	140.50 ± 22.41	1.073(0.311)	1.574(0.222)	5.052(0.034)
		Posttest	152.20 ± 14.58	136.82 ± 21.53			
		t(p)	−2.030(0.065)	1.081(0.303)			
PA-A (degree)	Non-dominant	Pretest	130.96 ± 21.51	128.32 ± 25.78	20.395(0.000)	0.927(0.346)	4.639(0.042)
		Posttest	149.58 ± 19.94	134.91 ± 26.60			
		t(p)	−4.517(0.001)	−1.774(0.104)			
	Dominant	Pretest	130.48 ± 30.72	126.74 ± 27.70	21.522(0.000)	1.642(0.213)	16.072(0.001)
		Posttest	151.93 ± 20.55	128.30 ± 29.63			
		t(p)	−4.964(0.000)	−0.722(0.485)			

Values expressed as mean ± standard deviation; FPRE—functional progressive resistive exercise; CG—control group; PA-P—popliteal angle in passive range of motion; PA-S—popliteal angle in speed range of motion; PA-A—popliteal angle in active range of motion.

3.5. Comparison of Dynamic Balance between the FPRE Group and the Control Group

Dynamic balance was assessed with the modified FRT in two different positions: forward reaching position and side reaching position. Statistically significant time factor effects were observed on the S-FRT ($p < 0.05$) and statistically significant time × group interaction effects were observed on the forward functional reach test (F-FRT) and side functional reach test (S-FRT) ($p < 0.05$).

A paired t-test revealed a statistically significant increase on the F-FRT and S-FRT in the FPRE group after the intervention ($p < 0.05$). However, in the control group, the mean value between the pre and posttest showed no significant difference (Table 6).

Table 6. Modified functional reach test (forward and side) ($N = 25$).

Balance		FPRE Group ($n = 13$)	CG Group ($n = 12$)	Time F(p)	Group F(p)	Time × Group F(p)
F-FRT (cm)	Pretest	21.62 ± 6.87	28.17 ± 14.49	0.842(0.368)	0.459(0.505)	10.259(0.004)
	Posttest	26.65 ± 7.92	25.37 ± 10.20			
	t(p)	−5.635(0.000)	1.186(0.261)			
S-FRT (cm)	Pretest	11.57 ± 5.72	15.52 ± 10.43	6.344(0.019)	0.408(0.529)	4.361(0.048)
	Posttest	16.21 ± 5.37	15.95 ± 8.266			
	t(p)	−3.734(0.003)	−0.270(0.793)			

Values expressed as mean ± standard deviation; FPRE—functional progressive resistance exercise; CG—control group; F-FRT—forward functional reach test; S-FRT—side functional reach test.

3.6. Comparisons of the GMFM Score between the FPRE Group and the Control Group

Functional ability was assessed with the GMFM-88. A paired t-test revealed a statistically significant increase on the GMFM score in the FPRE group after the intervention ($p < 0.05$). However, in the control group, the mean value between the pre and posttest showed no significant difference (Table 7).

Table 7. GMFM score: Pre and post training and changes ($N = 25$).

Gross Motor Function		FPRE Group ($n = 13$)	CG Group ($n = 12$)	Time $F(p)$	Group $F(p)$	Time × Group $F(p)$
GMFM score	Pretest	69.98 ± 21.55	68.15 ± 27.15	0.346(0.562)	0.288(0.597)	1.744(0.200)
	Posttest	71.78 ± 21.05	63.48 ± 27.48			
	$t(p)$	−2.696(0.019)	0.924(0.375)			

Values expressed as mean ± standard deviation; FPRE—functional progressive resistance exercise; CG—control group; GMFM—gross motor function measure.

4. Discussion

4.1. Knee Extensor Muscle Strength

CP affects physical activity and has a negative impact on the child's physical development. The spasticity and loss of strength experienced by children with CP results increased incidence of gait disorders and increased energy consumption in comparison with their healthy peers [9,37]. The muscle weakness in the lower extremity is particularly important for ambulation and requires strength training in children with CP [38]. Several studies have provided adequate evidence of a correlation between muscle strength and lower extremity function [39,40]. Indeed, increase in lower extremity muscle strength leads to positive effects on functional activities and flexibility [41].

In this study, FPRE strength training programs were used. Using the handheld dynamometer to examine the knee extensor strength, time factor effects were observed on the knee extensor muscle strength of the dominant side and non-dominant side ($p < 0.05$) and time × group interaction effects were observed on the knee extensor muscle strength of the dominant side ($p < 0.05$); these results are consistent with the results of previous studies, suggesting that strength training in CP leads to increased lower extremity strength [24]. The protocol for increasing muscle strength of the knee extensor in CP are numerous; however, due to the low methodological quality of previous studies, the effects of the study protocols may have been overestimated [42]. Nevertheless, we believe that organized method, resistance and repetitions of the exercises can increase lower extremity strength. Anttila et al. [43] reported that strengthen training in children with CP is not recommended, as it may increase spasticity, which can lead to reduction in range of motion—as well as difficulty with ambulation. However, recently increasing evidence and systemic reviews have shown that strength training can improve muscle strength in children with CP with no adverse effects on spasticity. These results indicate that FPRE training in CP leads to increased muscle power and lower extremity muscle strength in children with CP and could be considered for use in rehabilitation programs.

4.2. Structure of Quadriceps in Rehabilitative Ultrasound Imaging

RUSI uses USI to aid rehabilitation of neuromusculoskeletal disorders. Physical therapists have used RUSI to evaluate function and related soft tissue morphology and muscle during exercise and physical tasks [30]. Muscle cross-sectional area has a direct relationship with the capacity of muscle to produce power [7]. RUSI was used to assess thickness of the quadriceps and cross-sectional area of the rectus femoris in order to provide a clinical measurement of increased quadricep volume, which indicates increase of lower extremity strength [44].

In this study, changes in thickness and cross-sectional area of the quadriceps were assessed with RUSI. The time × group interaction effects ($p < 0.05$) were observed for TQ of the dominant and non-dominant sides and CSA of the dominant side. Lee et al. [45] performed progressive functional training on 26 children with CP with spasticity. For 6 weeks, neurodevelopmental treatment and FPRE were performed in the experimental group. The muscle thickness of the quadriceps femoris (QF), cross-sectional area of the rectus femoris (RF) and pennation angle of the gastrocnemius (GCM) were measured with RUSI, and results after the intervention showed significant improvement on those variables ($p < 0.05$). In the experimental group, QF thickness increased from 1.6 cm to 1.9 cm and RF

CSA increased from 1.2 cm^2 to 2.1 cm^2 [45]. Additionally, increase in structure-related measurements is strongly correlated with increased muscle strength [7].

The outcomes may result from the fact that motor units work in an inadequate, irregular and slower than normal manner following upper motor neuron damage. Therefore, the more affected side cannot activate as normal muscle [17,46]. Thus, it is difficult to generalize this information to all pediatric cases, since this study was not conducted among normally developing children; however, increments observed in the results indicate that FPRE protocol has a positive effect on increasing muscle strength in children with spastic CP.

4.3. Muscle Tone According to Popliteal Angle in Passive, Speed and Active Ranges of Motion

Individual spastic muscle fibers with increased tensile strength are stiffer than controls; therefore, to elongate a spastic muscle fiber, more force is needed [47]. Developments of contractures and passive stiffness could be the result of weakened agonist muscles that result in the inability of the spastic antagonist muscle to elongate, thereby perpetuating a pattern of weakness [48]. Popliteal angle was measured in passive, speed and active conditions to determine the impact of FPRE on muscle tone of the hamstring. The FPRE is an exercise program which allows the co-contraction of both quadriceps and hamstring, thereby increasing agonist muscle strength to enable elongation of the antagonist muscle to reduce muscle tone of the lower extremity and increase the popliteal angle.

In this study, popliteal angles in passive, speed and active ranges of motion were assessed in order to evaluate the effects of FPRE on lower leg range of motion and strength. Time × group interaction effects ($p < 0.05$) were observed for the PA-P, PA-S and PA-A of the dominant and non-dominant side. Results of studies by Stubbs, P.W et al. [49] and Scholtes, V.A., et al. [50] imply that muscle strengthening does not increase muscle tone. A prior study has shown that muscle tone was significantly lower after the intervention in the training group (median 1, 0/7; $p < 0.01$) and control group (median 0, 0/4; $p = 0.02$) after implementing a muscle strengthening exercise on children with CP and spasticity, p. A prior study on dynamic strength exercises of the knee extensor showed statistically significant changes (pre: 64.4 to post: 92.6) in the training group and (pre: 60.8 to post: 65.3) control group ($p < 0.05$) [49,50]. Generally, the muscle tension in children with CP develops due to elongated sarcomeres, with decreased action and myosin interaction, which limits the number of cross-bridges causing reduced force production capability [17]. This biomechanical disadvantage may disrupt the ability of the muscle to sufficiently contract to produce the required functional movement.

This study suggests that an increase in passive range of motion allows for adequate muscle length to produce maximum muscle contraction, which could be the reason for an increment in active range of motion. An increase in agonist muscle strength may be strongly correlated with increment in speed range of motion due to co-activation of the thigh muscle. This result provides valid evidence of the effect of FPRE, which can be used in the future to treat children with CP.

4.4. Dynamic Balance

A comparison of normally developing children-with-children with CP reveals that children with CP have delayed onset of postural muscle activity. In addition, there is a high level of co-activation of agonist and antagonist muscles at a joint and multiple muscle action sequences are impaired. This can cause difficulty in balance control in CP [4,51]. In this study, dynamic balance was examined using the FRT. An increase in lower extremity muscle strength was shown to be closely correlated with increased dynamic balance ability, which was assessed with the modified FRT [52].

In this study, dynamic balance was assessed with the modified functional reach test in two different positions: forward reaching position and side reaching position. Time effects were observed with the S-FRT ($p < 0.05$), while time × group interaction effects were observed with the F-FRT and S-FRT ($p < 0.05$). FPRE program comprises exercises such as sit to stand and side step-up with load. This exercise program includes voluntary co-contraction of both lower extremity muscles, quadriceps and hamstring muscles [53]. After performing the sit to stand exercise, the FRT value increased in the exercise group; results for the asymmetric paretic limb position in the control group were pre 19.36 ± 6.42 to post 23.43 ± 3.85, while in the training group results were pre 14.91 ± 6.11 to post 21.81 ± 4.59, which indicates that the training group showed statistical improvement after intervention t(p); −2.287(0.034) ($p < 0.05$).

In our FPRE study, the FRT was measured in two positions, position forward (F) reaching and side (S) reaching in the FPRE group. These results imply that the exercise protocol of the FPRE, which includes co-activation and functional strengthening, can have a positive effect on dynamic balance.

4.5. GMFM in Functional Ability

It is important to accurately measure changes in the acquisition of total motor skills to determine the impact on rehabilitation and the effectiveness of the intervention program in children with CP. The GMFM-88 is an effective measuring tool to detect changes in gross motor function in children with CP [35]. In spastic diplegia CP, strength was highly related to functional abilities [54].

In this study, functional ability was assessed with the GMFM-88. A paired *t*-test revealed a statistically significant increase after the intervention on the GMFM score in the FPRE group ($p < 0.05$).

Ross et al. [54] indicates that lower extremity strength has a strong correlation with functional ability. They conducted a study to determine the relationship between strength and GMFM-66 on CP. The study included 49 boys and 48 girls; mean age ± standard deviation, 9.11 ± 4.8 years. Aggregate strength consisting of values for the ankle dorsiflexors and plantar flexors, knee extensors and flexors and hip abductors and adductors averaged across sides was strongly correlated to the GMFM-66 (r.83). In this study, the GMFM-88 score of the FPRE group increased from a pre-mean value of 69.98 ± 21.55 to a post mean value of 71.78 ± 21.05, (0.019, $p < 0.05$) compared to the control group in which there was a reduction in the GMFM-88 score from 68.15 ± 27.15 to 63.48 ± 27.48 after the intervention. Although an increase was shown in the FPRE group, the change between the two groups was not statistically significant. This result may be due to the duration of the intervention. The results of the study conducted by Bryant et al. [55] indicate that a six-week program can show significant difference on GMFM-88D scores, but not on GMFM-66 or GMFM-88E scores.

The RUSI is an effective assessment device, which can successfully measure thickness and cross-sectional area of the quadriceps, which are associated with lower extremity strength [30]. Quadriceps thickness can also be an indicator of muscle strength, Ohata et al. [8] identified a relationship between thickness of the quadriceps and activity limitation in children and adolescents with CP. Muscle thickness of the quadriceps showed a significant correlation with the GMFM-66 score ($r = 0.52$, $p = 0.001$, 95% CI 0.24 to 0.72). This result suggests that lower extremity muscle thickness may be strongly correlated with functional ability of the child with CP.

This study has the following limitations: a short 6-week intervention period and a small sample size. This makes it difficult to generalize the findings to all children with CP. It is also difficult to control all the factors that may affect the child's activities of daily living.

5. Conclusions

Present study was conducted with twenty-five children to determine the effects of FPRE on strength, lower extremity structure, muscle tone, dynamic balance and functional ability in children with spastic cerebral palsy. This study confirmed that FPRE exerts a positive effect by increasing lower extremity strength and morphology of quadriceps muscle, reducing muscle tone and increasing dynamic balance and functional ability in children with spastic CP. Therefore, we suggest FPRE as an effective, safe and convenient intervention that can be implemented in a six-week period in children with CP in rehabilitation.

Author Contributions: Conceptualization, H.-J.C. and B.-H.L.; Data curation, H.-J.C.; Investigation, H.-J.C.; Methodology, H.-J.C.; Project administration, B.-H.L.; Supervision, B.-H.L.; Writing – original draft, H.-J.C.; Writing – review & editing, B.-H.L. All authors have read and agreed to the published version of the manuscript.

Funding: This study was supported by a grant from the NRF (NRF-2018R1D1A1B07045746), which is funded by the Korean government.

Conflicts of Interest: The authors declare no conflict of interest.

References

1. Richards, C.L.; Malouin, F. Cerebral palsy: Definition, assessment and rehabilitation. *Handb. Clin. Neurol.* **2013**, *111*, 83–95.
2. Green, L.B.; Hurvitz, E.A. Cerebral palsy. *Phys. Med. Rehabil. Clin. N. Am.* **2007**, *18*, 859–882. [CrossRef] [PubMed]
3. Himmelmann, K.; Uvebrant, P. The panorama of cerebral palsy in Sweden. XI. Changing patterns in the birth-year period 2003–2006. *Acta Paediatr.* **2014**, *103*, 618–624. [CrossRef]
4. Nashner, L.; Shumway-Cook, A.; Marin, O. Stance posture control in select groups of children with cerebral palsy: Deficits in sensory organization and muscular coordination. *Exp. Brain Res.* **1983**, *49*, 393–409. [CrossRef] [PubMed]
5. Braun, K.V.N.; Christensen, D.; Doernberg, N.; Schieve, L.; Rice, C.; Wiggins, L.; Schendel, D.; Yeargin-Allsopp, M. Trends in the Prevalence of Autism Spectrum Disorder, Cerebral Palsy, Hearing Loss, Intellectual Disability, and Vision Impairment, Metropolitan Atlanta, 1991–2010. *PLoS ONE* **2015**, *10*, e0124120. [CrossRef]
6. Lampe, R.; Grassl, S.; Mitternacht, J.; Gerdesmeyer, L.; Gradinger, R. MRT-measurements of muscle volumes of the lower extremities of youths with spastic hemiplegia caused by cerebral palsy. *Brain Dev.* **2006**, *28*, 500–506. [CrossRef]
7. Moreau, N.G.; Simpson, K.N.; Teefey, S.A.; Damiano, D.L. Muscle Architecture Predicts Maximum Strength and Is Related to Activity Levels in Cerebral Palsy. *Phys. Ther.* **2010**, *90*, 1619–1630. [CrossRef]
8. Ohata, K.; Tsuboyama, T.; Haruta, T.; Ichihashi, N.; Kato, T.; Nakamura, T. Relation between muscle thickness, spasticity, and activity limitations in children and adolescents with cerebral palsy. *Dev. Med. Child Neurol.* **2008**, *50*, 152–156. [CrossRef]
9. Aviram, R.; Harries, N.; Namourah, I.; Amro, A.; Bar-Haim, S. Effects of a group circuit progressive resistance training program compared with a treadmill training program for adolescents with cerebral palsy. *Dev. Neurorehabilit.* **2016**, *20*, 347–354. [CrossRef]
10. Hoffman, R.; Corr, B.B.; Stuberg, W.A.; Arpin, D.; Kurz, M.J. Changes in lower extremity strength may be related to the walking speed improvements in children with cerebral palsy after gait training. *Res. Dev. Disabil.* **2018**, *73*, 14–20. [CrossRef]
11. Fowler, E.G.; Kolobe, T.H.; Damiano, D.L.; Thorpe, D.E.; Morgan, D.W.; Brunstrom, J.E.; Coster, W.J.; Henderson, R.C.; Pitetti, K.H.; Rimmer, J.H.; et al. Promotion of Physical Fitness and Prevention of Secondary Conditions for Children With Cerebral Palsy: Section on Pediatrics Research Summit Proceedings. *Phys. Ther.* **2007**, *87*, 1495–1510. [CrossRef]
12. Miller, T.L. A hospital-based exercise program to improve body composition, strength, and abdominal adiposity in 2 HIV-infected children. *AIDS Read.* **2007**, *17*, 450–452.
13. Kelly, M.; Darrah, J. Aquatic exercise for children with cerebral palsy. *Dev. Med. Child Neurol.* **2005**, *47*, 838. [CrossRef]
14. Dunst, C.J. Research Foundations for Evidence-Informed Early Childhood Intervention Performance Checklists. *Educ. Sci.* **2017**, *7*, 78. [CrossRef]
15. Cameron, R.A.; Brousseau, J.; Cerracchio, K.; Clark, T.; Cotsalas, T.; Eisen, K.; Gannotti, M.E. Multimodal Community-Based Exercise for Children with Cerebral Palsy: Dosing Interventions for Effectiveness. *Crit. Rev. Phys. Rehabilit. Med.* **2018**, *30*, 15–43. [CrossRef]
16. Ozal, C.; Türker, D.; Korkem, D. Strength Training in People with Cerebral Palsy. *Cereb. Palsy Curr. Steps* **2016**, 103. [CrossRef]
17. Mockford, M.; Caulton, J.M. The Pathophysiological Basis of Weakness in Children With Cerebral Palsy. *Pediatr. Phys. Ther.* **2010**, *22*, 222–233. [CrossRef] [PubMed]
18. Clutterbuck, G.L.; Auld, M.; Johnston, L. Active exercise interventions improve gross motor function of ambulant/semi-ambulant children with cerebral palsy: A systematic review. *Disabil. Rehabilit.* **2018**, *41*, 1131–1151. [CrossRef]

19. Faigenbaum, A.D.; Kraemer, W.J.; Blimkie, C.J.R.; Jeffreys, I.; Micheli, L.J.; Nitka, M.; Rowland, T.W. Youth Resistance Training: Updated Position Statement Paper From the National Strength and Conditioning Association. *J. Strength Cond. Res.* **2009**, *23*, S60–S79. [CrossRef]
20. Damiano, D.L. Progressive resistance exercise increases strength but does not improve objective measures of mobility in young people with cerebral palsy. *J. Physiother.* **2014**, *60*, 58. [CrossRef]
21. Dos Santos, A.N.; Pavão, S.L.; Rocha, N. Sit-to-stand movement in children with cerebral palsy: A critical review. *Res. Dev. Disabil.* **2011**, *32*, 2243–2252. [CrossRef] [PubMed]
22. Mukherjee, A.; Chakravarty, A. Spasticity Mechanisms—For the Clinician. *Front. Neurol.* **2010**, *1*, 149. [CrossRef] [PubMed]
23. Palisano, R.; Rosenbaum, P.; Walter, S.; Russell, D.; Wood, E.; Galuppi, B. Development and reliability of a system to classify gross motor function in children with cerebral palsy. *Dev. Med. Child Neurol.* **1997**, *39*, 214–223. [CrossRef] [PubMed]
24. Scholtes, V.A.; Becher, J.G.; Janssen-Potten, Y.J.; Dekkers, H.; Smallenbroek, L.; Dallmeijer, A.J. Effectiveness of functional progressive resistance exercise training on walking ability in children with cerebral palsy: A randomized controlled trial. *Res. Dev. Disabil.* **2012**, *33*, 181–188. [CrossRef]
25. Dahab, K.S.; McCambridge, T.M. Strength Training in Children and Adolescents: Raising the Bar for Young Athletes? *Sports Health* **2009**, *1*, 223–226. [CrossRef]
26. Verschuren, O.; Ada, L.; Maltais, D.B.; Gorter, J.W.; Scianni, A.; Ketelaar, M. Muscle Strengthening in Children and Adolescents With Spastic Cerebral Palsy: Considerations for Future Resistance Training Protocols. *Phys. Ther.* **2011**, *91*, 1130–1139. [CrossRef]
27. Winter, D.A.; Wells, R.P.; Orr, G.W. Errors in the use of isokinetic dynamometers. *Eur. J. Appl. Physiol. Occup. Physiol.* **1981**, *46*, 397–408. [CrossRef]
28. Chesterton, L.S.; Sim, J.; Wright, C.C.; Foster, N.E. Interrater Reliability of Algometry in Measuring Pressure Pain Thresholds in Healthy Humans, Using Multiple Raters. *Clin. J. Pain* **2007**, *23*, 760–766. [CrossRef]
29. Teyhen, D.; Koppenhaver, S. Rehabilitative ultrasound imaging. *J. Physiother.* **2011**, *57*, 196. [CrossRef]
30. Fernández-Carnero, J.; Arias-Buría, J.L.; Zaldívar, J.N.C.; Quiñones, A.L.; Calvo-Lobo, C.; Martín-Saborido, C. Rehabilitative Ultrasound Imaging Evaluation in Physiotherapy: Piloting a Systematic Review. *Appl. Sci.* **2019**, *9*, 181. [CrossRef]
31. Sarikaya, I.A.; Inan, M.; Seker, A. Improvement of popliteal angle with semitendinosus or gastrocnemius tenotomies in children with cerebral palsy. *Acta Orthop. Traumatol. Turc.* **2015**, *49*, 51–56. [CrossRef] [PubMed]
32. Domínguez, G.; Cardiel, E.; Arias, S.; Rogeli, P. A Digital Goniometer Based on Encoders for Measuring Knee-Joint Position in An Orthosis. In Proceedings of the 2013 World Congress on Nature and Biologically Inspired Computing, Fargo, ND, USA, 12–14 August 2013.
33. Duncan, P.W.; Weiner, D.K.; Chandler, J.; Studenski, S. Functional Reach: A New Clinical Measure of Balance. *J. Gerontol.* **1990**, *45*, M192–M197. [CrossRef] [PubMed]
34. Mason, A.N.; Lum, J.; Milligan, A.; Robinson, J. Functional Reach Test. *Crit. Rev. Phys. Rehabilit. Med.* **2018**, *30*, 105–107. [CrossRef]
35. Alotaibi, M.; Long, T.; Kennedy, E.; Bavishi, S. The efficacy of GMFM-88 and GMFM-66 to detect changes in gross motor function in children with cerebral palsy (CP): A literature review. *Disabil. Rehabil.* **2013**, *36*, 617–627. [CrossRef]
36. Lee, J.H.; Lim, H.K.; Park, E.; Song, J.; Lee, H.S.; Ko, J.; Kim, M. Reliability and Applicability of the Bayley Scale of Infant Development-II for Children With Cerebral Palsy. *Ann. Rehabilit. Med.* **2013**, *37*, 167–174. [CrossRef]
37. Orlin, M.N.; Palisano, R.J.; Chiarello, L.A.; Kang, L.-J.; Polansky, M.; Almasri, N.; Maggs, J. Participation in home, extracurricular, and community activities among children and young people with cerebral palsy. *Dev. Med. Child Neurol.* **2009**, *52*, 160–166. [CrossRef]
38. Wiley, M.E.; Damiano, D.L. Lower-extremity strength profiles in spastic cerebral palsy. *Dev. Med. Child Neurol.* **1998**, *40*, 100–107. [CrossRef]
39. Lee, J.H.; Sung, I.Y.; Yoo, J.Y. Therapeutic effects of strengthening exercise on gait function of cerebral palsy. *Disabil. Rehabilit.* **2008**, *30*, 1439–1444. [CrossRef]

40. Liao, H.-F.; Liu, Y.-C.; Liu, W.-Y.; Lin, Y.-T. Effectiveness of Loaded Sit-to-Stand Resistance Exercise for Children With Mild Spastic Diplegia: A Randomized Clinical Trial. *Arch. Phys. Med. Rehabilit.* **2007**, *88*, 25–31. [CrossRef]
41. McBurney, H.; Taylor, N.F.; Dodd, K.J.; Graham, H.K. A qualitative analysis of the benefits of strength training for young people with cerebral palsy. *Dev. Med. Child Neurol.* **2003**, *45*, 658–663. [CrossRef]
42. Dodd, K.J.; Taylor, N.F.; Damiano, D.L. A systematic review of the effectiveness of strength-training programs for people with cerebral palsy. *Arch. Phys. Med. Rehabilit.* **2002**, *83*, 1157–1164. [CrossRef]
43. Anttila, H.; Autti-Rämö, I.; Suoranta, J.; Mäkelä, M.; Malmivaara, A. Effectiveness of physical therapy interventions for children with cerebral palsy: A systematic review. *BMC Pediatr.* **2008**, *8*, 14. [CrossRef] [PubMed]
44. Ramírez-Fuentes, C.; Mínguez-Blasco, P.; Ostiz, F.; Sánchez-Rodríguez, D.; Messaggi-Sartor, M.; Macías, R.; Muniesa, J.M.; Rodríguez, D.A.; Vila, J.; Perkisas, S.; et al. Ultrasound assessment of rectus femoris muscle in rehabilitation patients with chronic obstructive pulmonary disease screened for sarcopenia: Correlation of muscle size with quadriceps strength and fat-free mass. *Eur. Geriatr. Med.* **2018**, *10*, 89–97. [CrossRef] [PubMed]
45. Lee, M.; Ko, Y.; Shin, M.M.S.; Lee, W. The effects of progressive functional training on lower limb muscle architecture and motor function in children with spastic cerebral palsy. *J. Phys. Ther. Sci.* **2015**, *27*, 1581–1584. [CrossRef] [PubMed]
46. Rose, J.; McGill, K.C. Neuromuscular activation and motor-unit firing characteristics in cerebral palsy. *Dev. Med. Child Neurol.* **2005**, *47*, 329–336. [CrossRef]
47. Fridén, J.; Lieber, R.L. Spastic muscle cells are shorter and stiffer than normal cells. *Muscle Nerve* **2003**, *27*, 157–164. [CrossRef]
48. Toner, L.V.; Cook, K.; Elder, G.C.B. Improved ankle function in children with cerebral palsy after computer-assisted motor learning. *Dev. Med. Child Neurol.* **1998**, *40*, 829–835. [CrossRef]
49. Stubbs, P.W.; Diong, J. The effect of strengthening interventions on strength and physical performance in people with cerebral palsy (PEDro synthesis). *Br. J. Sports Med.* **2016**, *50*, 189–190. [CrossRef]
50. Scholtes, V.A.; Dallmeijer, A.J.; Rameckers, E.; Verschuren, O.; Tempelaars, E.; Hensen, M.; Becher, J.G. Lower limb strength training in children with cerebral palsy—A randomized controlled trial protocol for functional strength training based on progressive resistance exercise principles. *BMC Pediatr.* **2008**, *8*, 41. [CrossRef]
51. Burtner, P.; Qualls, C.; Woollacott, M. Muscle activation characteristics of stance balance control in children with spastic cerebral palsy. *Gait Posture* **1998**, *8*, 163–174. [CrossRef]
52. Saquetto, M.; Carvalho, V.; Silva, C.; Conceição, C.; Gomes-Neto, M. The effects of whole body vibration on mobility and balance in children with cerebral palsy: A systematic review with meta-analysis. *J. Musculoskelet. Neuronal Interact.* **2015**, *15*, 137–144. [PubMed]
53. Ross, S.M.; Macdonald, M.; Bigouette, J.P. Effects of strength training on mobility in adults with cerebral palsy: A systematic review. *Disabil. Health J.* **2016**, *9*, 375–384. [CrossRef] [PubMed]
54. Ross, S.A.; Engsberg, J.R. Relationships between Spasticity, Strength, Gait, and the GMFM-66 in Persons With Spastic Diplegia Cerebral Palsy. *Arch. Phys. Med. Rehabilit.* **2007**, *88*, 1114–1120. [CrossRef] [PubMed]
55. Bryant, E.C.; Pountney, T.; Williams, H.; Edelman, N. Can a six-week exercise intervention improve gross motor function for non-ambulant children with cerebral palsy? A pilot randomized controlled trial. *Clin. Rehabilit.* **2012**, *27*, 150–159. [CrossRef] [PubMed]

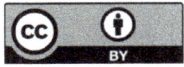

© 2020 by the authors. Licensee MDPI, Basel, Switzerland. This article is an open access article distributed under the terms and conditions of the Creative Commons Attribution (CC BY) license (http://creativecommons.org/licenses/by/4.0/).

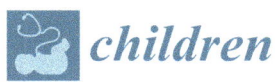

Article

Effect of Action Observation Training on Spasticity, Gross Motor Function, and Balance in Children with Diplegia Cerebral Palsy

Young-a Jeong [1] and Byoung-Hee Lee [2,*]

1. Graduate School of Physical Therapy, Sahmyook University, Seoul 01795, Korea; nay5130@naver.com
2. Department of Physical Therapy, Sahmyook University, Seoul 01795, Korea
* Correspondence: 3679@syu.ac.kr; Tel.: +82-2-3399-1634

Received: 11 May 2020; Accepted: 16 June 2020; Published: 18 June 2020

Abstract: This study evaluated the effect of action observation training on spasticity, gross motor function, and balance in children with spastic diplegia cerebral palsy. Eighteen children with cerebral palsy participated in this study. The participants were randomized into the action observation training group ($n = 9$) and a control group ($n = 9$). The action observation training group repeatedly practiced the action with their motor skills, while the control group practiced conventional physical therapy. Both groups received 30 min sessions, 3 days a week, for 6 weeks. To confirm the effects of intervention, the spasticity, gross motor function measurement (GMFM), and pediatric reaching test (PRT) were evaluated. The results showed that in the plantar flexor contracture test of both sides, the Modified Tardieu Scale (MTS) of the right side of knee joints, GMFM-B, C, and D were significantly increased between pre- and post-intervention within both groups ($p < 0.05$). PRT was significantly increased between pre- and post-intervention within the both groups ($p < 0.05$), and there was a significant difference between the two groups ($p < 0.05$). These results suggest that action observation training is both feasible and beneficial for improving spasticity, gross motor function, and balance in children with spastic diplegia cerebral palsy.

Keywords: cerebral palsy; action observation; spasticity; gross motor function; balance

1. Introduction

Cerebral palsy is a non-progressive disorder that affects the development of the brain of fetuses or infants, and presents as limited activity, movement, and postural disorders [1]. Stiff diplegia is a disorder that shows more dysfunction in the lower extremities than the upper extremities [2], while spasticity diplegia is characterized by ununiformed abnormal movements, unstable continuous movements, and large patterns of motion [3]. Cerebral palsy also leads to limits in balance due to muscle weakness in skeletal muscles, excessive reflexes, simultaneous contraction of agonist and antagonist muscles, delayed response of the ankle muscles, and shrink posture [4].

Balance is important for most functional skill movements; this includes the integration of sensory inputs to structure the body's perception of the center of gravity, and perform appropriate musculoskeletal responses to unexpected movements or to stabilize during moments of instability [4]. However, in cerebral palsy, when balance is affected, it increases compensation usage of the upper extremities, which is followed by restricted movement of the upper limbs. This may cause limitation in the function of the upper extremities [5], performance, and learning activities of daily life, as well as problems in movement and a limitation of social roles and community participation [6].

Spasticity means intermittent or persistently involuntary disordered sensory motor control caused by upper motor neuron lesions [7]. Prolonged spasticity causes abnormal posture, limitation of movement, and limitation and construction of active or passive joint movement [8]. In order to improve the spasticity and balance in children with cerebral palsy, various treatment intervention methods have been used; these include botulinum toxin injection [9,10], anticipatory postural adjustments [11], dynamic ankle-foot orthosis [12], whole-body vibration [13], and extracorporeal shock wave therapy [14]. Recently, a new method of treating upper limb motor deficits using action observation training has been proposed for patients with stroke [15,16] and cerebral palsy [17–19]. Action observation training is a cognitive intervention technique that is used to improve and learn exercise skills in sports athletes, the general public, and patients with motor impairments. This training involves using the activity of mirror neurons with excitement characteristics when actually exercising or watching others perform tasks [16]. Various studies on movement observation training have been proposed, but most relate to restoring the upper limb function of stroke and cerebral palsy patients, and studies on the spasticity, gross motor function, and balance in cerebral palsy for movement observation training are insufficient. Therefore, this study aims to contribute to the improvement of rehabilitation in children with spastic diplegia cerebral palsy by verifying the effect of action observation training on the treatment of spasticity, gross motor function, and balance.

2. Materials and Methods

The participants of this study were selected from 30 children who were diagnosed with diplegia cerebral palsy and undergoing physical therapy at K-hospital and E-center in Seoul. The specific selection criteria of the study subjects were children between 5 and 11 years old diagnosed with diplegic cerebral palsy, without visual impairment and visual field defects, able to follow the researcher's instructions, GMFCS (gross motor function classification system) level I–III, and with ankle dorsal flexors and plantar flexors better than poor + in manual muscle test. The parents of the children consented to their participation in this study after the purpose of the study was explained and they were informed that they could withdraw at any time. The exclusion criteria included children with a modified assessment scale (MAS) of 2 or more, children who have not had a seizure in the last 6 months, or those who received botulinum injections 6 months prior to the study. This study was conducted with the approval of the Research Institutional Review Board of Sahmyook University. The objective and the procedures to be performed in the study were fully understood by the subjects, and all participants' parents provided informed consent for inclusion in the study. Therefore, this study was based on the ethical principles of the Declaration of Helsinki.

The past history of the 30 children who agreed to the study was examined, and other orthopedic or neurological examinations were performed by the attending doctor before treatment. Of the 30 children at K-hospital, 3 children were under GMFCS level III and 1 child had a seizure within the past 6 months. A total of 22 patients were selected, with the exception of 2 with communication disorders and 2 children who had received botulinum injection 6 months prior. The selected 22 children were divided into either the action observation training group (AOT) at K-hospital or the control group E-center, which is a cerebral palsy treatment center nearby K-hospital for the blind, and each group included 11 participants. All subjects picked a go stone with black or white stone from a box containing 22 pieces of stone. The action observation training program was conducted three times a week for 30 min, for a total of 18 times, and general physical therapy was given 5 times/week for 30 min for a total of 6 weeks. One week before training and 1 week after training proceeded the evaluation. In the AOT, two children who could not participate in the experiment due to personal reasons and seizure dropped out of the control group, and two children who could not participate in the experiment due to personal reasons dropped out. Finally, each group included 9 children, and a total of 18 children were included in the experiment.

2.1. Action Observation Training

In this study, action observation training (AOT) focused on spasticity of lower extremities, contracture, gross motor function measurement (GMFM), and balance ability. Children with cerebral palsy watched a video on a 42-inch screen, installed 1 m in front of their chairs, while sitting comfortably with their arms resting, but they were not allowed to physically follow the video or move. The model of the video's motion observation exercise was performed by a therapist who treated the child, and the training video consists of 4 stages that varied by difficulty, and the video of each step was watched for the entire week. The participants watched a video of a task presented by a therapist, and after completing the assignment, they performed the steps, if a step was too difficult to perform, retraining was conducted. The first stage consisted of movements to improve balance in the sitting position, the second stage consisted of sit-to-stand movements, the third stage consisted of standing movements to improve balance, and the fourth stage consisted of walking sideways (Table 1). The viewing time was 15 min, and 5 min of physical training was conducted with the therapist based on the content of the video, after 5 min of watching. In order to enhance the effectiveness of the action observation training, the participants watched the video at a designated time in a quiet place without noise. The children were instructed to concentrate on the video for 1 min intervals to allow for the attention span of children. Entire experiments were conducted by the same investigator from the beginning to the end of the experiment.

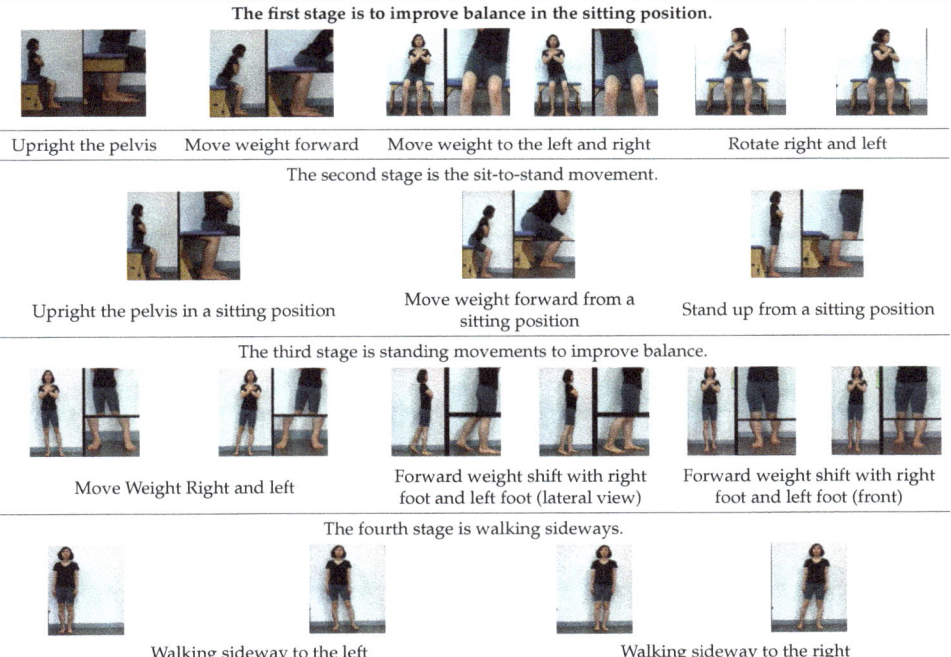

Table 1. Action observation training protocol.

2.2. General Physical Therapy

Neurodevelopment treatment is a 1:1 treatment between a patient and therapist. The participants received 6 weeks of general physical therapy, 5 times a week, for 30 min each session, according to the treatment schedule of the hospital. The exercise program included lying to sitting position, moving in the sitting posture, sitting and standing up, posture training for learning a normal gait pattern, weight bearing and weight movement training in the straight posture, walking training on the flat floor, and stair walking.

2.3. Outcome Measurements

2.3.1. Spasticity of Ankle Joint

In this study, changes in the spasticity was used; ankle stiffness and Modified Tardieu Scale. An electronic joint goniometer (Gemred, China, 2014) was used to measure the ankle stiffness. In the supine position, the examiner extended the knee joint and examined the ankle stiffness in a relaxed state without muscle contraction. After the subject's heel fixed and dorsi-flexion with manual force as much as possible, it was maintained for 4 s in the end range. A Modified Tardieu Scale (MTS) was used to measure the muscle spasticity; the reliability for children with cerebral palsy was ICC = 0.54–0.95, which is defined as a high reliability [17]. The Tardieu scale can measure muscle spasticity by testing the response of the muscle to stretch at three types of velocity (i.e., slow as possible, speed of the limb segment when falling, and as fast as possible).

2.3.2. Gross Motor Function

The gross motor function measure-88(GMFM) is a tool for measuring and recording changes in an exercise level over time or as a result of treatment; the scores are ordinal on a 4-point grade scale after observing the movements of children with cerebral palsy. The evaluation items were composed of the following: A scale, lying and rolling position with 17 items; B scale, 20 items in the sitting position; C scale, 14 items in the standing position of the instrument and knees; D scale, 13 items in the standing position; and E scale, 24 items, including walking, running, and jumping activities. In cerebral palsy children, the inter-evaluator reliability was ICC = 0.929 and the test-retest reliability was ICC = 0.92–0.99 [18]. The results were compared using the sitting posture (B scale), device and knee standing posture (C scale), standing posture (D scale), and walking, running, and leap activity (E scale).

2.3.3. Balance Function Measurement

The pediatric arm stretch test is a modified version of the functional reach test (FRT) with forward stretch and side stretch in a sitting position. The test-retest reliability of cerebral palsy children was $r = 0.54$–0.88 and the inter-tester reliability $r = 0.50$–0.93 [19]. The side and forward distances of children from the sitting position were measured before and after intervention.

2.3.4. Data Analyses

SPSS ver. 21.0 was used to calculate the mean and standard deviation. The normality of variables was tested using the Shapiro–Wilks test, and all variables were normally distributed. General characteristics of the subjects were provided as descriptive statistics, and independent t-tests were conducted to identify the differences among the groups. Paired t-tests were conducted before and after the action observation training. Statistical significance was assumed when $p < 0.05$.

3. Results

The characteristics of the 18 participants who completed the experiment are shown in Table 2. No differences in gender, age, height, weight, GMFCS level were detected between the two groups at baseline.

Table 2. General characteristics of subjects ($N = 18$).

Parameters	AOT ($n = 9$)	Control ($n = 9$)	t (p)
Gender, M/F (n, %)	3 (33.3)/6 (66.7)	5 (55.0)/4 (45.0)	1.141 (0.270)
Age (years)	7.44 ± 1.88 [a]	6.90 ± 1.79	0.646 (0.527)
Height (cm)	122.60 ± 13.86	123.24 ± 14.18	−0.099 (0.922)
Weight (kg)	23.01 ± 6.71	27.73 ± 10.19	−1.176 (0.256)
GMFCS (I/II/III)	4/2/3	4/3/2	0.210 (0.837)

[a] Mean ± SD; AOT: Action observation training; GMFCS: Gross motor function classification system.

3.1. Spasticity of Ankle Joint

Changes in the spasticity of the study subjects in the two groups were as follows (Table 3). In the right ankle stiffness test, the AOT increased by 6.58° ($p < 0.05$), from 4.00° before training to 10.58° after training, the control group increased significantly by 4.39° and there was no significant difference between the two groups. In the left ankle joint examination of MTS, the AOT showed a significant increase of 6.10° ($p < 0.05$), and the control group showed a significant increase of 4.38° ($p < 0.05$) and there was no significant difference between the two groups. In the evaluation of spasticity right knee joint of MTS, the AOT showed a significant decrease of 2.91° ($p < 0.05$), and the control group showed a significant decrease of 1.09° ($p < 0.05$) and there was no significant difference between the two groups. In the left knee joint MTS evaluation, the AOT showed a significant decrease of 1.86° ($p < 0.05$), while the control group showed no significant difference and there was significant difference between the two groups ($p < 0.05$).

Table 3. Differences in spasticity of ankle joint ($N = 18$).

Parameters		AOT ($n = 9$)	Control ($n = 9$)	t (p)
Ankle stiffness-right side (°)	Before	4.00 ± 4.72 [a]	3.77 ± 4.87	−1.651 (0.118)
	After	10.58 ± 3.36	8.16 ± 3.58	
	Before-after	−6.58 ± 2.46	−4.39 ± 3.12	
	t(p)	−8.018 (0.000)	−4.223 (0.003)	
Ankle stiffness-left side (°)	Before	3.40 ± 4.92	3.34 ± 4.13	−1.411 (0.177)
	After	9.50 ± 3.45	7.71 ± 2.98	
	Before-after	−6.10 ± 2.76	−4.38 ± 2.41	
	t(p)	−6.632 (0.000)	−5.439 (0.001)	
MTS-right (kg)	Before	4.78 ± 3.26	3.57 ± 3.35	1.325 (0.204)
	After	2.91 ± 2.53	2.47 ± 2.99	
	Before-after	1.87 ± 1.46	1.09 ± 0.98	
	t(p)	−4.987 (0.001)	3.335 (0.010)	
MTS-left (kg)	Before	3.77 ± 1.46	4.29 ± 3.19	2.236 (0.040)
	After	1.91 ± 1.20	3.94 ± 3.28	
	Before-after	1.86 ± 1.80	0.34 ± 0.93	
	t(p)	3.093 (0.015)	1.106 (0.301)	

[a] Mean ± SD; AOT: Action observation training; MTS: Modified Tardieu Scale.

3.2. Gross Motor Function

Table 4 shows the changes in the GMFM before and after the intervention. The mean of the GMFM-B items of AOT showed a significantly increased by 5.12%, from 93.33% before training to 98.45% after training ($p < 0.05$), and the control group was significantly increased by 1.85% ($p < 0.05$), and there was no significant difference between the two groups. The mean of the GMFM-C items significantly increased by 6.56% ($p < 0.05$) in the AOT, and the control group also significantly increased by 2.89% ($p < 0.05$), but there was no significant difference between the two groups. Finally, the mean of the GMFM-E items of the AOT showed a significantly increased by 6.51% ($p < 0.05$), and there was significant difference between the two groups ($p < 0.05$).

3.3. Balance Function Measurement

The change in dynamic balance between the two groups is shown in Table 5. The right side stretching average of the children's arm stretch test of AOT was significantly increased by 3.28 cm ($p < 0.05$), and the control group also significantly increased by 1.40 cm, and there was a significant difference between the two groups ($p < 0.05$). The left side stretching average of the AOT significantly increased by 4.08 cm ($p < 0.05$), and that of the control group significantly increased by 1.42 cm ($p < 0.05$) and there was a significant difference between the two groups ($p < 0.05$). The average of the right forward extension of the pediatric extension test significantly increased by 4.60 cm, and the control group significantly increased by 2.02 cm ($p < 0.05$) and there was a significant difference between the two groups ($p < 0.05$). The average of the left forward stretching of the AOT significantly increased by 4.25 cm ($p < 0.05$), while the average of the control group significantly increased by 2.04 cm ($p < 0.05$) and there was a significant difference between the two groups ($p < 0.05$).

Table 4. Differences in gross motor function ($N = 18$).

Parameters		AOT ($n = 9$)	Control ($n = 9$)	t (p)
GMFM-B (%)	Before	93.33 ± 6.07 [a]	93.89 ± 5.40	−1.991 (0.064)
	After	98.45 ± 2.34	95.74 ± 4.72	
	Before-after	−5.12 ± 4.60	−1.85 ± 1.76	
	t(p)	−3.339 (0.010)	−3.162 (0.013)	
GMFM-C (%)	Before	88.36 ± 10.68	89.94 ± 9.88	−1.737 (0.102)
	After	94.92 ± 5.89	91.83 ± 8.49	
	Before-after	−6.56 ± 5.28	−2.89 ± 3.53	
	t(p)	−3.731 (0.006)	−2.449 (0.040)	
GMFM-D (%)	Before	60.68 ± 29.79	68.94 ± 23.02	−1.928 (0.072)
	After	77.48 ± 20.61	75.78 ± 21.79	
	Before-after	−16.80 ± 12.76	−6.84 ± 8.79	
	t(p)	−3.949 (0.004)	−2.334 (0.048)	
GMFM-E (%)	Before	46.26 ± 38.00	50.30 ± 32.82	−3.583 (0.002)
	After	52.77 ± 37.93	51.54 ± 32.26	
	Before-after	−6.51 ± 4.11	−1.23 ± 1.62	
	t(p)	−4.752 (0.001)	−2.285 (0.052)	

[a] Mean ± SD; AOT: Action observation training; GMFM: Gross motor function measure.

Table 5. Differences in balance function ($N = 18$).

Parameters		AOT ($n = 9$)	Control ($n = 9$)	t (p)
PRT lateral-right (cm)	Before	15.52 ± 6.12 [a]	14.94 ± 6.21	−2.327 (0.033)
	After	18.80 ± 6.42	16.33 ± 6.87	
	Before-after	−3.28 ± 1.71	−1.40 ± 1.72	
	t(p)	−5.751 (0.000)	−2.433 (0.041)	
PRT lateral-left (cm)	Before	14.34 ± 5.17	14.96 ± 6.68	−3.551 (0.003)
	After	18.42 ± 5.27	16.37 ± 6.75	
	Before-after	−4.08 ± 1.52	−1.42 ± 1.65	
	t(p)	−8.022 (0.000)	−2.578 (0.033)	
PRT frontal-right (cm)	Before	22.78 ± 7.16	20.35 ± 7.64	−2.154 (0.047)
	After	27.38 ± 7.81	22.37 ± 6.79	
	Before-after	−4.60 ± 2.87	−2.02 ± 2.16	
	t(p)	−4.811 (0.001)	−2.803 (0.023)	
PRT frontal-left (cm)	Before	22.60 ± 7.58	19.86 ± 7.54	−2.339 (0.033)
	After	26.85 ± 7.19	21.90 ± 7.41	
	Before-after	−4.25 ± 2.05	−2.04 ± 1.96	
	t(p)	−6.213 (0.000)	−3.116 (0.014)	

[a] Mean ± SD; AOT: Action observation training; PRT: Pediatric reaching test.

4. Discussion

Spasticity is the most common feature of cerebral palsy and occurs in approximately 85% of children with cerebral palsy, and correct assessment and treatment of spasticity are considered important. [20]. Most children with cerebral palsy spasticity have an asymmetrical body and disordered balance, leading to difficulties in daily activities [21]. In this study, changes in spasticity before and after training were confirmed by an ankle joint test and knee joint MTS. Curtis et al. (2014) [22] used an interactive dynamical stander to study low lateral flexor muscle spasticity of the ankle in children with cerebral palsy. Six children with cerebral palsy aged 4–10 years who were GMFCS level I–III were trained to activate ankle dorsi flexion for 10 weeks through ankle movements of the interactive dynamic stander of computer games. As a result, it was noted that the median active and passive dorsi flexion of the ankle increased by 5° and 10°, respectively; therefore, this training could function as a new clinical conservative treatment of ankle flexion in cerebral palsy children. In the right ankle joint contraction test in spasticity of ankle joint, both groups had a significant increase from before training to after training ($p < 0.05$), and in the left ankle joint contraction test, the AOT and control group increased from before training to after training ($p < 0.05$). Both groups' range of motion of ankle was significantly increased because of symmetrical weight-bearing during the intervention and its stimulation of proprioceptive sensibility. Improvement in the range of motion of the ankle, which is a functional ankle movement, is possibly due to the voluntary forward, backward, left, and right weight shift movements of the lower extremity during the stage 1 to 3 in AOT. Increase in the range of motion of the ankle in the control group and the exercise program included sitting and standing up, weight-bearing, and weight movement training in the straight posture.

In the MTS used to examine the degree of spasticity, the right knee joint of the action observation training participants was 4.78° before training and 2.91° after training. The knee joint decreased from 3.77° before training to 1.91° after training, which is consistent with the results of previous studies and suggests that there is a connection between construction and rigidity. These results indicate that the range of motion of the ankle joint is increased with regards to ankle construction, and the action observation training program images provide the children to simultaneously watch the full-motion images and the enlarged images of the movements, which are an important part of the joint's movement, were shown enlarged of children with diplegic cerebral palsy.

GMFM-88 is used as a most common tool to evaluate the function of children with cerebral palsy and down's syndrome [23] by measuring and recording changes in exercise levels over time or over treatment outcomes [24]. In the current study, the B scale of the AOT was 93.33% before training and 98.45% after training, the C scale was 88.36% before training and 94.92% after training, the D scale was 60.68% before training and 77.48% after training, and the E scale was 46.26% before training and 52.77% after training. There was a significant difference before and after training ($p < 0.05$), and also in the B scale, C scale, D scale, and E scale in the control group ($p < 0.05$). This was supported by the results of the AOT group in this study since a more significant change in the GMFM-E results was observed compared to the control group. Although conducted in a relatively short amount of time, the repeated viewing of the videos (including shifting the body weight forward and backward), standing movements to improve balance in the third stage, and walking sideways in the fourth stage allowed for an easier understanding of the specific positions for each action and their order. This increased the exercise's learning effects.

Park et al. reported [25] the effects of horseback riding treatment on gross motor function and functional performance in children with stiff cerebral palsy, and demonstrated a significant difference between the experimental group and the control group. Mahasup et al. studied [26] the effects of motor observation on 30 children with stiff diplegia cerebral palsy by applying action observation training for 2 months. In total, 15 control groups received general physical therapy that included the Bobath concept once a week, and 15 experimental groups performed action observation training three times a day; they demonstrated a significant difference in running and running and jumping between the two groups. The results of the current study are in agreement with previous studies and confirm that action observation training shows positive effects in improving GMFM. Therefore, action observation training improves the function of participants according to exercise level, and the action observation training was considered to contribute to the improvement of daily life skills and mobility of spastic bilateral lower limbs in cerebral palsy.

Children with cerebral palsy often have difficulty with sitting posture balance and have unstable postures, such as asymmetrical trunks and bending [27]. In addition, children with cerebral palsy have reduced movements in the trunk, pelvis, and lower extremities, so they stand and walk in unprepared condition, raising the upper extremities or excessively extending the upper bodies to compensate for insufficient antigravity activity [28]. Auld and Johnston (2014) [29] investigated the effects of an

8-week local community-based strengthening and balance exercise group on exercise in children with cerebral palsy. Five children with spastic diplegia cerebral palsy and five children with hemiplegia cerebral palsy participated in the study, and the results demonstrated that the participants' balance ability increased significantly in Movement Assessment Battery for Children and anterior and lateral extension ($p < 0.05$). In the current study, the right side stretch of the AOT increased from 15.52 cm before training to 18.8 cm after training, the left side of the side stretch increased from 14.34 cm before training to 18.42 cm after training, the right side of the forward stretch increased from 22.78 cm before training to 27.38 cm after training, and the left side of the forward stretch increased from 22.6 cm before training to 26.85 cm after the training. The improvement of the arm stretch test indicates an improvement in balance, and it is thought that the movement observation training contributed to uniform weight bearing, postural alignment, and the ability to change direction by improving the muscles. There was also a significant difference before and after training in the two groups ($p < 0.05$); this may be due to the effect of action observation training on brain activity in the primary motor area, and the activation of cognitive activities related to motor memory formation and understanding of other people's behavior through imitation [30].

This study has the following limitations: this study has a short 6-week intervention period, and this study comprises a small sample size. This makes it difficult to generalize the findings to all children with CP. It is also difficult to control all of the factors that might affect the child's hormones affect because of puberty, scoliosis or hip problems, any influence of bracing on knee or ankle range of motion and spasticity, and activities of daily living. Furthermore, several of the participants had a short attention span while concentrating on the action observation, making it difficult for the treatment to last long as planned. This could be explained by the fact that children with spastic CP are not only impaired by the regulation ability of the muscular system and sensory deprivation, but are also deprived of cognitive function [31]. This study confirmed that action observation training has shown positive effects in improving the spasticity of ankle joint, gross motor function, and balance in children with cerebral palsy.

Author Contributions: Conceptualization, Y.-a.J., and B.-H.L.; Data curation, Y.-a.J.; Methodology, Y.-a.J., and B.-H.L.; Project administration, B.-H.L.; Supervision, B.-H.L.; Visualization, Y.-a.J.; Writing–original draft, Y.-a.J.; Writing–review & editing, B.-H.L. All authors have read and agreed to the published version of the manuscript.

Funding: This study was supported by a grant from the NRF (NRF-2018R1D1A1B07045746), which is funded by the Korean government.

Conflicts of Interest: The authors declare no conflict of interest.

References

1. Bax, M.; Goldstein, M.; Rosenbaum, P.; Leviton, A.; Paneth, N.; Dan, B.; Jacobsson, B.; Damiano, D. Executive Committee for the Definition of Cerebral Palsy. Proposed definition and classification of cerebral palsy, April 2005. *Dev. Med. Child Neurol.* **2005**, *47*, 571–576. [CrossRef] [PubMed]
2. Schwartz, M.H.; Viehweger, E.; Stout, J.; Novacheck, T.F.; Gage, J.R. Comprehensive treatment of ambulatory children with cerebral palsy: An outcome assessment. *J. Pediatr. Orthop.* **2004**, *24*, 45–53. [CrossRef]
3. Yokochi, K. Motor functions in non-ambulatory children with spastic diplegia and periventricular leukomalacia. *Brain Dev.* **2001**, *23*, 327–332. [CrossRef]
4. Woollacott, M.H.; Shumway-Cook, A. Postural dysfunction during standing and walking in children with cerebral palsy: What are the underlying problems and what new therapies might improve balance? *Neural Plast.* **2005**, *12*, 211–219; discussion 63–72. [CrossRef] [PubMed]
5. Case-Smith, J. Parenting a child with a chronic medical condition. *Am. J. Occup. Ther.* **2004**, *58*, 551–560. [CrossRef]
6. Yonetsu, R.; Iwata, A.; Surya, J.; Unase, K.; Shimizu, J. Sit-to-stand movement changes in preschool-aged children with spastic diplegia following one neurodevelopmental treatment session—A pilot study. *Disabil. Rehabil.* **2015**, *37*, 1643–1650. [CrossRef]

7. Trompetto, C.; Marinelli, L.; Mori, L.; Pelosin, E.; Curra, A.; Molfetta, L.; Abbruzzese, G. Pathophysiology of spasticity: Implications for neurorehabilitation. *Biomed. Res. Int.* **2014**, *2014*, 354906. [CrossRef]
8. Bani-Ahmed, A. The evidence for prolonged muscle stretching in ankle joint management in upper motor neuron lesions: Considerations for rehabilitation - a systematic review. *Top Stroke Rehabil.* **2019**, *26*, 153–161. [CrossRef]
9. Multani, I.; Manji, J.; Hastings-Ison, T.; Khot, A.; Graham, K. Botulinum Toxin in the Management of Children with Cerebral Palsy. *Paediatr. Drugs* **2019**, *21*, 261–281. [CrossRef] [PubMed]
10. Ross Raftemo, A.E.; Mahendran, A.; Hollung, S.J.; Jahnsen, R.B.; Lydersen, S.; Vik, T.; Andersen, G.L. Use of botulinum toxin A in children with cerebral palsy. *Tidsskr. Nor. Laegeforen.* **2019**, *139*, 8.
11. Shiratori, T.; Girolami, G.L.; Aruin, A.S. Anticipatory postural adjustments associated with a loading perturbation in children with hemiplegic and diplegic cerebral palsy. *Exp. Brain Res.* **2016**, *234*, 2967–2978. [CrossRef] [PubMed]
12. Lintanf, M.; Bourseul, J.S.; Houx, L.; Lempereur, M.; Brochard, S.; Pons, C. Effect of ankle-foot orthoses on gait, balance and gross motor function in children with cerebral palsy: A systematic review and meta-analysis. *Clin. Rehabil.* **2018**, *32*, 1175–1188. [CrossRef]
13. Pin, T.W.; Butler, P.B.; Purves, S. Use of whole body vibration therapy in individuals with moderate severity of cerebral palsy- a feasibility study. *BMC Neurol.* **2019**, *19*, 80. [CrossRef] [PubMed]
14. Lin, Y.; Wang, G.; Wang, B. Rehabilitation treatment of spastic cerebral palsy with radial extracorporeal shock wave therapy and rehabilitation therapy. *Med. (Baltim.)* **2018**, *97*, e13828. [CrossRef] [PubMed]
15. Zhang, B.; Kan, L.; Dong, A.; Zhang, J.; Bai, Z.; Xie, Y.; Liu, Q.; Peng, Y. The effects of action observation training on improving upper limb motor functions in people with stroke: A systematic review and meta-analysis. *PLoS ONE* **2019**, *14*, e0221166. [CrossRef] [PubMed]
16. Kim, J.H.; Lee, B.H. Action observation training for functional activities after stroke: A pilot randomized controlled trial. *Neuro Rehabil.* **2013**, *33*, 565–574. [CrossRef] [PubMed]
17. Simon-Martinez, C.; Mailleux, L.; Ortibus, E.; Fehrenbach, A.; Sgandurra, G.; Cioni, G.; Desloovere, K.; Wenderoth, N.; Demaerel, P.; Sunaert, S.; et al. Combining constraint-induced movement therapy and action-observation training in children with unilateral cerebral palsy: A randomized controlled trial. *BMC Pediatr.* **2018**, *18*, 250. [CrossRef]
18. Buccino, G.; Molinaro, A.; Ambrosi, C.; Arisi, D.; Mascaro, L.; Pinardi, C.; Rossi, A.; Gasparotti, R.; Fazzi, E.; Galli, J. Action Observation Treatment Improves Upper Limb Motor Functions in Children with Cerebral Palsy: A Combined Clinical and Brain Imaging Study. *Neural. Plast.* **2018**, *2018*, 4843985. [CrossRef]
19. Sgandurra, G.; Cecchi, F.; Beani, E.; Mannari, I.; Maselli, M.; Falotico, F.P.; Inguaggiato, E.; Perazza, S.; Sicola, E.; Feys, H.; et al. Tele-UPCAT: Study protocol of a randomised controlled trial of a home-based Tele-monitored UPper limb Children Action observation Training for participants with unilateral cerebral palsy. *BMJ Open* **2018**, *8*, e017819.
20. Leonard, G.; Tremblay, F. Corticomotor facilitation associated with observation, imagery and imitation of hand actions: A comparative study in young and old adults. *Exp. Brain Res.* **2007**, *177*, 167–175. [CrossRef]
21. Numanoglu, A.; Gunel, M.K. Intraobserver reliability of modified Ashworth scale and modified Tardieu scale in the assessment of spasticity in children with cerebral palsy. *Acta Orthop. Traumatol. Turc.* **2012**, *46*, 196–200. [CrossRef]
22. Ko, J.; Kim, M. Reliability and responsiveness of the gross motor function measure-88 in children with cerebral palsy. *Phys. Ther.* **2013**, *93*, 393–400. [CrossRef] [PubMed]
23. Bartlett, D.; Birmingham, T. Validity and reliability of a pediatric reach test. *Pediatr. Phys. Ther.* **2003**, *15*, 84–92. [CrossRef] [PubMed]
24. Surveillance of cerebral palsy in Europe. A collaboration of cerebral palsy surveys and registers. Surveillance of Cerebral Palsy in Europe (SCPE). *Dev. Med. Child Neurol.* **2000**, *42*, 816–824. [CrossRef] [PubMed]
25. Lemmens, R.J.; Janssen-Potten, Y.J.; Timmermans, A.A.; Defesche, A.; Smeets, R.J.; Seelen, H.A. Arm hand skilled performance in cerebral palsy: Activity preferences and their movement components. *BMC Neurol.* **2014**, *14*, 52. [CrossRef]
26. Curtis, D.J.; Bencke, J.; Mygind, B. The effect of training in an interactive dynamic stander on ankle dorsiflexion and gross motor function in children with cerebral palsy. *Dev. Neurorehabil.* **2014**, *17*, 393–397. [CrossRef]

27. Tieman, B.L.; Palisano, R.J.; Gracely, E.J.; Rosenbaum, P.L. Gross motor capability and performance of mobility in children with cerebral palsy: A comparison across home, school, and outdoors/community settings. *Phys. Ther.* **2004**, *84*, 419–429. [CrossRef]
28. Damiano, D.L.; Abel, M.F. Relation of gait analysis to gross motor function in cerebral palsy. *Dev. Med. Child Neurol.* **1996**, *38*, 389–396. [CrossRef]
29. Park, E.S.; Rha, D.W.; Shin, J.S.; Kim, S.; Jung, S. Effects of hippotherapy on gross motor function and functional performance of children with cerebral palsy. *Yonsei Med. J.* **2014**, *55*, 1736–1742. [CrossRef]
30. Mahasup, N.; Sritipsukho, P.; Lekskulchai, R.; Hansakunachai, T. Effects of mirror neurons stimulation on motor skill rehabilitation in children with cerebral palsy: A clinical trial. *J. Med. Assoc. Thai.* **2012**, *95*, S166–S172.
31. Chan, G.; Miller, F. Assessment and treatment of children with cerebral palsy. *Orthop. Clin. N. Am.* **2014**, *45*, 313–325. [CrossRef] [PubMed]

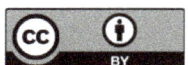

© 2020 by the authors. Licensee MDPI, Basel, Switzerland. This article is an open access article distributed under the terms and conditions of the Creative Commons Attribution (CC BY) license (http://creativecommons.org/licenses/by/4.0/).

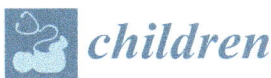

Review

Cognitive Assessment and Rehabilitation for Pediatric-Onset Multiple Sclerosis: A Scoping Review

Wei-Sheng Lin [1,*,†], Shan-Ju Lin [2,†] and Ting-Rong Hsu [1,3,4]

1. Department of Pediatrics, Taipei Veterans General Hospital, Taipei 11217, Taiwan; romberg@gmail.com
2. Department of Physical Medicine and Rehabilitation, National Taiwan University Hospital Yunlin Branch, Yunlin 640, Taiwan; y00964@ms1.ylh.gov.tw
3. Institute of Clinical Medicine, National Yang-Ming University, Taipei 112, Taiwan
4. Faculty of Medicine, National Yang-Ming University, Taipei 112, Taiwan
* Correspondence: wshenq@yahoo.com.tw
† These authors contributed equally to this work.

Received: 17 September 2020; Accepted: 10 October 2020; Published: 15 October 2020

Abstract: Cognitive impairment is increasingly recognized as an important clinical issue in pediatric multiple sclerosis (MS). However, variations regarding its assessment and remediation are noted in clinical arena. This scoping review aims to collate available evidence concerning cognitive assessment tool and cognitive rehabilitation for pediatric MS. We performed a systematic search of electronic databases (MEDLINE, PubMed, CINAHL Plus, and Web of Science) from inception to February 2020. Reference lists of included articles and trial registers were also searched. We included original studies published in English that addressed cognitive assessment tools or cognitive rehabilitation for pediatric-onset MS. Fourteen studies fulfilled our inclusion criteria. Among them, 11 studies evaluated the psychometric aspects of various cognitive assessment tools in the context of pediatric MS, and different neuro-cognitive domains were emphasized across studies. There were only three pilot studies reporting cognitive rehabilitation for pediatric-onset MS, all of which used home-based computerized programs targeting working memory and attention, respectively. Overall, more systematic research on cognitive assessment tools and rehabilitation for pediatric MS is needed to inform evidence-based practice. Computer-assisted cognitive assessment and rehabilitation appear feasible and deserve further studies.

Keywords: cognition; cognitive rehabilitation; pediatric multiple sclerosis

1. Introduction

Multiple sclerosis (MS) is a chronic central nervous system disorder characterized by inflammatory demyelination and neurodegeneration, and around 3–5% of patients have their disease onset prior to adulthood. Although physical disability is rarely seen in the first decade of disease course in pediatric-onset MS (POMS) [1], cognitive impairment is fairly common in this patient population. Findings across studies showed that around one-third of pediatric MS patients suffer from some degree of cognitive impairment, and it could be detected as early as nearing disease onset in a subset of patients [2–5]. Multiple cognitive domains have been reported to be affected in pediatric MS, including information processing speed, attention, working memory (WM), verbal and visuospatial memory, executive function, visuo-motor integration, and aspects of language function [4–10]. While reports of cognitive profiles of POMS have been accumulating, direct comparisons between these studies are often hampered by differences in patient characteristics and assessment tools. Indeed, it was noted that the results of cognitive evaluation might vary with the instruments used. For instance, Wuerfel et al. used several tests to tap WM and found that only more cognitively demanding tasks revealed group-level difference in WM performance between POMS and controls [6]. This exemplifies the importance to clarify the applicability and performance of various cognitive assessment tools in this patient population.

Despite growing awareness of cognitive issues in pediatric MS in recent years, there has been limited information to date concerning ways of cognitive remediation for these patients. Rehabilitative strategies for POMS are often extrapolated from those for adult MS in the real-world situations, but this approach needs validation. To obtain a panorama of this emerging field, we here seek to collate existing evidence on cognitive assessment tools and cognitive rehabilitation for POMS, which may serve as the basis for future directions of research and clinical practice.

2. Materials and Methods

We followed the methodological framework developed by Arksey and O'Malley [11], and this scoping review adheres to the Preferred Reporting Items for Systematic Reviews and Meta-analyses Extension for Scoping Reviews (PRISMA-ScR, Supplementary File S1) [12]. This study was retrospectively registered at Open Science Framework database (https://osf.io/uyd2q/) on 12 April 2020, and the review protocol is presented in Supplementary File S2.

2.1. Literature Search, Screening, and Selection

We conducted systematic literature searches in the following databases: PubMed, MEDLINE, CINAHL Plus, and Web of Science. Date of publication was not restricted (from inception to February 2020). The terms used in the searches were: "multiple sclerosis" AND ("pediatric" or "paediatric") AND ("cognitive" or "cognition"). The most recent search was executed on 21 March 2020. The titles and abstracts of retrieved articles were then screened for relevance to cognitive evaluation and/or cognitive rehabilitation. The inclusion criteria were: (a) peer-reviewed original studies published in English; (b) studies that specifically addressed either cognitive assessment tools or cognitive rehabilitation for POMS. The exclusion criteria were: (a) articles that were either not peer-reviewed (e.g., book chapter) or not reporting original studies (e.g., review paper); (b) studies that aimed to characterize the cognitive profile of POMS, rather than to examine the performance and applicability of cognitive assessment tools or the effects of cognitive rehabilitation in this patient population. Every effort was made to obtain the full text of all potentially relevant articles, which were examined to determine the eligibility. We also screened the reference lists of relevant articles. The above process was independently carried out by two of the authors (W.-S.L. and S.-J.L.), and discrepancies were resolved by discussion with the senior author (T.-R.H.) and consensus among the authors.

On the other hand, we also searched ClinicalTrials.gov, European Union Clinical Trials Register, and Open Science Framework database for trials or projects pertinent to the themes of our review.

2.2. Data Charting

The included articles were read by two of the authors (W.-S.L. and S.-J.L.), and relevant data were charted and tabulated. For studies evaluating cognitive assessment tools, we extracted the year of publication, the tests (and subtests, if applicable) of interest and their targeted cognitive domains, the characteristics of study participants (such as sample size of disease and control groups, demographic and disease-related features), and main findings (particularly in relation to psychometric performance). For studies evaluating cognitive rehabilitation, we extracted the mode of intervention (including its frequency and duration, requirement of supervision, and targeted cognitive domains), study design, the characteristics of study participants, effects of intervention (including effects on targeted and non-targeted domains, and sustainability of effect), and factors associated with outcomes.

For relevant clinical trials identified from trial registers, the principal investigator, the aim and the design of the trial, and other relevant information were collected.

3. Results

3.1. Original Studies Evaluating Cognitive Assessment Tools for Pediatric MS

The workflow of this scoping review is shown in Figure 1. We identified eleven original papers evaluating the performance of cognitive assessment tools in the context of pediatric MS, with the earliest one published in 2009 [13]. A summary of these articles is provided in Table 1. These studies were largely cross-sectional in design. They were either single- or multi-centric, and all were carried out in North America and Europe. The focus of these studies differed from one another. Some studies tried to establish normative data using regression-based approach [14–16], in which age-squared variable could be incorporated to better model the nonlinear quality of cognitive development [15,16]. Others investigated the performance of various cognitive assessment tools through comparisons between patients and healthy controls [7,13,15–21]. Among these, two studies aimed to construct batteries by picking up three to four tests with better discriminating abilities, and evaluated the performance of these batteries as screening tools [13,21]. Participants' satisfaction with the test was quantitatively reported in a study [17]. One study examined the interrelationships between tests tapping different cognitive domains [8]. A recurring finding yielded by these studies was the significant role of age and educational level in cognitive task performance in pediatric populations [14,17,21]. For instance, the symbol digit modalities test (SDMT) performance steadily improves with age in healthy children (8–17 years) [17]. On the other hand, older age predicted poorer SDMT performance in POMS after adjustment for disease severity (i.e., the expanded disability status scale, EDSS) [18]. Together these suggest divergent cognitive trajectories between normal children and pediatric patients with MS.

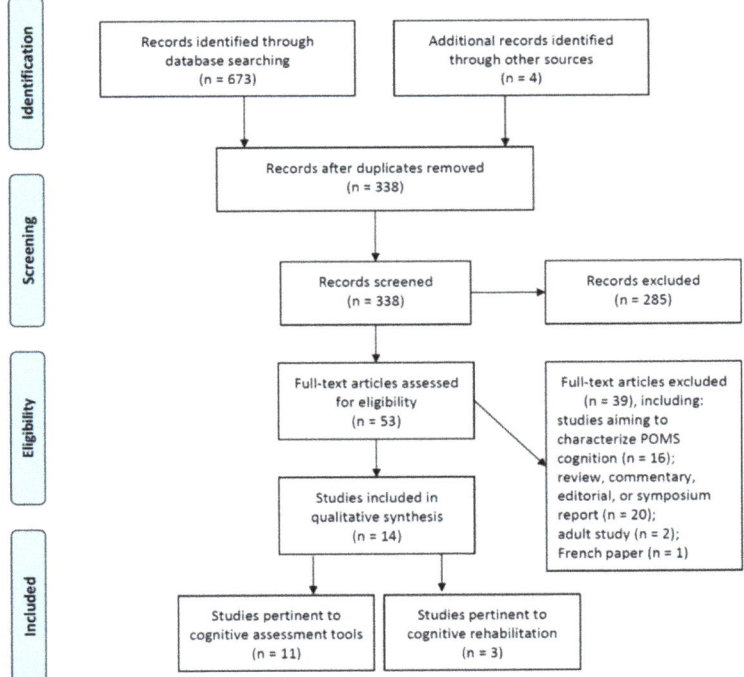

Figure 1. Diagram showing the workflow of literature search and selection process.

Table 1. Overview of studies evaluating instruments for cognitive assessment for pediatric-onset multiple sclerosis (POMS).

Author (Year)	Test/Battery	Participants	Subtests and Targeted Cognitive Domains	Main Findings and/or Additional Notes
Portaccio et al. (2009) [13]	Brief Neuropsychological Battery for Children (BNBC)	61 POMS (age 8.8–17.9 years), 58 matched HC	• WISC vocabulary: language • SDMT: processing speed, attention • TMT: processing speed, attention, executive function • SRT: verbal learning/memory	• Sensitivity: 96%, specificity: 76% (cut-off: failure on at least one test) • ~30 min
Smerbeck et al. (2011) [15]	Brief Visuospatial Memory Test–Revised (BVMTR)	51 POMS, 4 with ADEM, 92 HC (age 6–17)	• visuospatial learning/memory	• Regression-based pediatric norms • Significantly poorer performance in pediatric patients with demyelinating disorders, with medium and large effect size for BVMTR (Cohen's d −0.38~−0.71) and SDMT (Cohen's d −1.30) respectively, between children with demyelinating disorders and HC.
	SDMT (oral version)	22 POMS, 3 with ADEM, 92 HC (age 6–17)	• processing speed, attention	
Smerbeck et al. (2011) [20]	Brief Visuospatial Memory Test–revised (BVMTR)	43 POMS (age 9–18), 43 HC (age 9–18)	• visuospatial learning/memory	• significant difference between groups (Cohen's d 0.9)
	SDMT (oral version)	20 POMS (age 9–18), 20 HC (age 8–18)	• processing speed, attention	• significant difference between groups (Cohen's d 0.69)
Smerbeck et al. (2012) [16]	National MS Society Consensus Neuropsychological Battery for Pediatric Multiple Sclerosis (NBPMS)	51 POMS (age 9–18), 102 HC (age 5–18)	• WASI: intelligence • Grooved Pegboard Test: sensorimotor • EOWPVT: language • DKEFS Verbal Fluency: language • Beery–Buktenika Test of Visual-Motor Integration: visuospatial processing • CVLT-C: verbal learning/memory • CPT-II: executive function, attention • WISC-IV Digit Span: working memory • WISC-IV Coding B: processing speed, attention • Contingency Naming Test: executive function • DKEFS TMT: executive function	• Manual-based and regression-based (demographically adjusted) pediatric norms correlated strongly ($r > 0.7$) for all 30 variables. • In 19 out of 30 variables, regression-based norms more readily detected neuropsychological impairment in POMS.

Table 1. Cont.

Author (Year)	Test/Battery	Participants	Subtests and Targeted Cognitive Domains	Main Findings and/or Additional Notes
Charvet et al. (2014) [18]	Symbol Digit Modalities Test (SDMT, oral version)	70 POMS (70 underwent SDMT, 31 underwent neuropsychological testing), 40 other pediatric neurological diagnoses, 32 HC (note: significant difference in racial distribution between MS and HC)	• processing speed, attention	• SDMT showed 77% sensitivity and 81% specificity for neuropsychological impairment when the latter was done within one year, 100% sensitivity when the latter was done within two months. • SDMT z score was significantly correlated with neuropsychological evaluation aggregate z score ($r = 0.62$, $p < 0.001$). • Impaired SDMT performance in 37% of POMS and 9% of HC.
Bigi et al. (2017) [17]	Computer-Based Symbol Digit Modalities Test (c-SDMT)	27 POMS (22 female, 81.5%), age 8–18 years), 478 HC (237 female, 49.5%)	• processing speed, attention	• Regression analysis showed that increasing age (in the range 8–17) was significantly associated with better performance in HC. • High test–retest reliability (ICC = 0.91) in HC. • Total time to complete the task did not differ between POMS and HC, but POMS patients were less likely to show successively better performance over latter part of the task. • Over 85% of participants (HC and POMS) indicated that they liked the test.
Charvet et al. (2018) [19]	Brief International Cognitive Assessment for Multiple Sclerosis battery (BICAMS)	69 POMS (7–21 years), 66 HC (8–21 years)	• SDMT: processing speed, attention • BVMTR: visuospatial learning/memory • RAVLT: verbal learning/memory	• Specificity: 91% • Detection rate of cognitive impairment: 26% • ~15 min
	Cogstate Brief Battery	67 POMS, 48 HC	Three speeded processing tasks: • Detection: processing speed • Identification: attention • One-Back: working memory	• Specificity: 92% • Detection rate of cognitive impairment: 27% • Detection and identification tasks (but not one-back) significantly discriminated between POMS and HC. • ~15 min • BICAMS and Cogstate agreed in the classification of impairment in 74% of the full sample (69% and 85% agreement for POMS and HC, respectively).

Table 1. Cont.

Author (Year)	Test/Battery	Participants	Subtests and Targeted Cognitive Domains	Main Findings and/or Additional Notes
Kapanci et al. (2019) [8]	See subtests column (the study examined the interrelationships of tests tapping processing speed, working memory, and intelligence)	21 POMS, 21 matched HC	• Reaction time task: processing speed • Working memory task: working memory • Cattell's Culture Fair Test: intelligence	• Intelligence measured by Cattell's Culture Fair Test was significantly lower in POMS compared to HC. • 33% of the variance in psychometric intelligence between POMS and HC was explained by differences in RT task performance. • No difference in WM task performance between POMS and HC.
Brenton et al. (2019) [7]	See subtests column	20 POMS, 40 matched HC	• SDMT: processing speed, attention • PASAT (as a component of Multiple Sclerosis Functional Composite): processing speed, attention, working memory	• POMS patients performed significantly lower on SDMT ($p = 0.0002$) and PASAT ($p = 0.004$). • No significant correlation between SDMT z score and EDSS.
Falco et al. (2019) [14]	Rao's Brief Repeatable Battery (BRB)	76 HC (age 14–17)	• SRT and SRT-D: verbal learning/memory • SPART and SPART-D: visuospatial learning/memory • SDMT: processing speed, attention • PASAT: processing speed, attention, working memory • WLG: language (verbal fluency), executive function	• Regression analysis showed that gender, age, and education were important variables in adolescent population. • Younger age, male gender, and educational attainment were individually associated with better performance on SPART and SPART-D. • Male gender was also associated with better performance on PASAT.
Storm Van's Gravesande et al. (2019) [21]	Multiple Sclerosis Inventory of Cognition for Adolescents (MUSICADO)	106 POMS (age 12–18 years), 210 HC	• Phonemic verbal fluency task (RWT "s-words"): executive function, language (verbal fluency) • TMT-A: processing speed, attention • Digit Span Forward: working memory	• The phonemic verbal fluency task (RWT "s-words"), TMT-A, and Digit Span Forward tasks discriminated significantly between POMS and HC ($p < 0.001$, respectively). • Specificity of MUSICADO: 88.6% • Failure rate in POMS: RWT "s-words" 24.5%; TMT-A 17.9%, Digit Span Forward 15.1%.

Abbreviations: ADEM, acute disseminated encephalomyelitis; BICAMS, brief international cognitive assessment for multiple sclerosis battery; BVMTR, brief visuospatial memory test–revised; CPT-II, Conner's continuous performance test—second edition; CVLT-C, California verbal learning test for children; DKEFS, Delis-Kaplan executive function system; EDSS, expanded disability status scale; EOWPVT, expressive one word picture vocabulary test; HC, healthy controls; ICC, intraclass correlation coefficient; PASAT, paced auditory serial addition test; POMS, pediatric-onset multiple sclerosis; RAVLT, Rey auditory verbal learning test; RT, reaction time; RWT, Regensburger Wortflüssigkeitstest; SDMT, symbol digit modalities test; SPART, spatial recall test; SPART-D, SPART delayed recall; SRT, selective reminding test; SRT-D, SRT delayed recall; TMT, trail-making test; WASI, Wechsler abbreviated scales of intelligence; WISC-IV, Wechsler intelligence scale for children—fourth edition; WLG, word list generation; WM, working memory.

3.2. Original Studies Evaluating Cognitive Rehabilitation for POMS

We identified three original studies evaluating the effects of cognitive rehabilitation for POMS [22–24]. Their study design was summarized in Table 2. All three studies comprised interventions using home-based, computerized cognitive training. The targeted cognitive domains were working memory [22,23] and attention [24], respectively. The duration of a single training session was similar across these studies (45 min to 1 h), while the intensity varies from twice to five times per week. These studies were all pilot and exploratory in nature. The sample size was small (5–16 patients) and was not preplanned based on power analysis. No healthy control group was included in these studies. The study on attention retraining was a double-blind randomized clinical trial, using nonspecific training as the comparator arm. There was no comparator arm in the other two studies, hence the role of practice effect in neuropsychological evaluation cannot be clarified. The outcome measures included not only targeted cognitive function but also more extensive neuropsychological performance [23,24], and aspects of feasibility (adherence and tolerance to the training program) were evaluated as the main outcome in one study [23].

The results of these studies were summarized in Table 3. The study on attention retraining showed not only positive effects on attention and related cognitive domains, but also far transfer effect on visuospatial memory [24]. On the other hand, the other two studies, both focusing on working memory training, showed only modest effect on objective working memory measures, at group level. The far transfer effect was either inconspicuous [23] or not assessed [22] in these two studies. Hubacher et al. demonstrated that the training effect was sustained for nine months in both responders [22]. The sustainability of training effect was not assessed in the other two studies. Reported factors associated with outcomes of cognitive rehabilitation include various measures of disease burden, normalized brain volume, and general intelligence [22,23]. These are generally in line with the theory of brain reserve and cognitive reserve [25].

3.3. Registered Clinical Trials Primarily Focusing on Cognitive Issues in POMS

We searched on ClinicalTrials.gov, European Union Clinical Trials Register, and Open Science Framework database for pertinent trials or projects on 4 March 2020. Only three trials were considered most relevant. One trial aimed to explore the electrophysiological mechanisms underlying cognitive dysfunction in pediatric MS. The other was a randomized controlled trial assessing the efficacy of a home-based computerized program for retraining attention in pediatric patients with MS. These two trials were completed, and the results of the latter one has been published and included in the present review [24]. The third one is an ongoing randomized clinical trial aiming to assess the cognitive impact of a virtual reality videogame exercise program. More information about these trials is summarized in Table 4.

Table 2. Overview of studies evaluating cognitive rehabilitation for POMS: Study design.

Author (Year)	Intervention (Duration and Frequency)	Supervision or Coaching	Targeted Cognitive Domain	Study Participants	Comparator Group	Outcome Measures
Hubacher et al. (2015) [22]	computerized training (BrainStim) for 4 weeks (45 min/session, 4 times/week)	supervised by a psychologist once per week	working memory (visuospatial and verbal)	5 juvenile MS patients (age 12–17 years; 3 females)	Absent	Cognitive measures: working memory (visuospatial and verbal) and attention (alertness)
Simone et al. (2018) [24]	computerized training for 3 months (1 h/session, twice/week)	a psychologist called patients every week and met patients and their caregiver/parent every month	attention	16 POMS patients (age 15.75 ± 1.74 years; 9 females)	Present (nonspecific training)	Neuropsychological performance (using elaborate test battery)
Till et al. (2019) [23]	web-based training (Cogmed™) for 5 weeks (<1 h/session, 5 d/week)	weekly telephone support by a trained Cogmed™ Coach	working memory (visuospatial and verbal)	9 POMS patients (age 19.3 ± 4.1 years; 6 females)	Absent	Feasibility measures: adherence and tolerance; Cognitive measures: working memory, processing speed, visuospatial judgment

Table 3. Original studies evaluating cognitive rehabilitation for POMS: Summary of results.

Author (Year)	Intervention	Effects on Targeted or Related Cognitive Domains	Far Transfer Effect	Sustainability of Effect	Factors Associated with Training Response, and Additional Notes
Hubacher et al. (2015) [22]	computerized training (BrainStim) for 4 weeks (45 min/session, 4 times/week)	Two (of 5) were responders; both responders showed better WM (visuospatial and verbal), processing speed, and alertness.	Not assessed	Sustained behavioral response at 9 months in both responders	Disease activity and general intelligence may be factors associated with training response.
Simone et al. (2018) [24]	computerized training for 3 months (1 h/session, twice/week)	Improved attention, processing speed, and WM.	Improved executive function and visuospatial memory	NA	Not reported
Till et al. (2019) [23]	web-based training (Cogmed™) for 5 weeks (<1 h/session, 5 d/week)	Subjective: 8 (out of 9) reported improvement in WM; Objective: medium to large effect size on neuropsychological measures of WM.	Limited	NA	Indicators of feasibility: 6/9 adherence; 8/9 tolerance. The participant who showed the least improvement had the youngest age at disease onset, longest disease duration, highest number of relapses, and lowest normalized brain volume. The participant who did not tolerate the training had the lowest IQ.

Abbreviations: NA, not available; WM: working memory.

Table 4. Registered clinical trials primarily focusing on cognitive issues in POMS.

ClinicalTrials.Gov Identifier	NCT03066752	NCT03190902	NCT03933020
Aim	To study the neural mechanisms underlying cognitive dysfunction	To assess the efficacy of a computerized program for retraining attention	To assess the cognitive impact of a home-based virtual reality videogame exercise program
Study period	March~November 2017	September 2015~April 2016	May 2019~June 2020
Study type	Observational	Interventional	Interventional
Trial design	Prospective case-control	Double blind, randomized clinical trial	Single blind, randomized clinical trial
Ages eligible for study	6–18 years	up to 17 years	15–25 years
Recruitment status	Completed	Completed	Recruiting
Enrollment	10 cases, 10 controls (actual)	8 cases, 8 controls (actual)	12 cases, 12 controls (estimated)
Principal investigator	E. Ann Yeh	Pietro Iaffaldano	Stephanie Garcia-Tarodo

4. Discussions

Cognitive issues in pediatric MS have become a research priority in this field, and more studies surrounding cognitive evaluation for these patients were published over the past decade. Although routine cognitive screening is recommended for pediatric MS [26], and cognition has been incorporated into disease activity measure and treatment consideration [5,27,28], the best assessment tools for pediatric MS remain to be determined. Findings yielded by commonly used tools were sometimes discrepant across studies. For instance, SDMT has been recommended and widely used as a screening tool in adult and pediatric MS [26,29], whereas its sensitivity in pediatric MS was occasionally challenged [17,21,30,31], particularly in early stage of the disease. Brief international cognitive assessment for multiple sclerosis (BICAMS) and a Cogstate brief battery were shown to exhibit comparable sensitivity in detecting cognitive impairment in POMS [19]. These two batteries were subsequently employed in a study investigating the neuroanatomical correlates of cognitive impairment in POMS; however, the findings cast doubt on the discriminative power of BICAMS [31]. Trail making test (TMT)-B performance more readily differentiated between POMS and controls compared to TMT-A in earlier studies [13,30], whereas the reverse was found in later studies [21,32]. Bartlett et al. reported that verbal memory as assessed by Rey auditory verbal learning test (RAVLT) was impaired in POMS [31], while Storm Van's Gravesande et al. found no significant verbal memory deficit in POMS using Verbaler Lern- und Merkfähigkeitstest (the German version of RAVLT) [21]. Discrepant results were also reported with regard to visuospatial memory tapped by brief visuospatial memory test-revised (BVMTR) versus Rey–Osterrieth figure tests [15,21]. Collectively, these reports underscore the need for more systematic evaluation on the selection and performance of neuropsychological tests in pediatric patients with MS.

Some of the discrepancies mentioned above could be due to differences in patient characteristics across studies. For example, the average EDSS score of subjects involved in evaluating multiple sclerosis inventory of cognition for adolescents (MUSICADO) was only 0.65, which might explain why verbal and visuospatial memory were preserved in POMS compared to controls in that study [21]. Indeed, Amato et al. reported that differences in verbal and visuospatial memory performance between POMS and healthy controls were inconspicuous at baseline [30], yet became significant at five-year follow-up [9]. Given that psychometric properties could be disease stage-dependent, and floor or ceiling effects could occur, longitudinal studies may be required to delineate the performance of various assessment tools along the disease course. This dimension has been less addressed so far, and existing studies were mostly cross-sectional in design.

Another issue concerns the validation of cognitive assessment tools in different populations and language versions, as was being performed for application of BICAMS in adults [33,34]. This is particularly important for pediatric populations, as many of the cognitive assessment tools have been shown to be age-sensitive during preteen to adolescent periods [14,15,17,21], and the relationship between age and cognitive development may be nonlinear [16]. In addition, most of existing studies were performed in North America and Europe, where some ethnic groups may be underrepresented [15]. Therefore, validation of the tools, including establishment of the norms, remain to be carried out in different populations.

Fatigue is relatively common in POMS, and it could be an important confounder for executive function or other aspects of cognitive performance in these patients [21,30,35–38]. Fatigue also poses practical limitation on the duration of assessment for these patients. It is intriguing to note that in the study evaluating computerized version of SDMT, POMS patients exhibited an "inverted U" pattern of performance over successive trials, in contrast to the progressive improvement observed in healthy controls [17]. This suggests a time-on-task effect, a psychological construct related to cognitive fatigue, which was often investigated using questionnaire [21,35]. A psychometric analysis of time-on-task effect in pediatric MS patients using cognitive tests involving repeated tasks (such as reaction time tasks) may deserve further research, as it could provide a complementary indicator of cognitive fatigue. The intra-individual variability, another neuropsychological metric of white matter pathology, could also be explored using these tasks [39]. Overall, more studies are needed to clarify whether and how fatigue and cognitive performance interact in pediatric MS.

On the other hand, our review shows that dedicated studies concerning cognitive rehabilitation for POMS remain scarce. A search for relevant clinical trials (Table 4) also showed a paucity of research specifically focusing on cognitive issues for pediatric MS, though this could be an underestimation because some trials may be retrospectively registered. Most current trials of cognitive rehabilitation for MS aim exclusively at adult populations [40,41]. We identified only three published studies evaluating effects of cognitive rehabilitation for POMS, two of which aimed to improve working memory and one targeted attention [22–24]. It is remarkable that all of these studies used home-based computerized programs. Although group- or institution-based rehabilitation may have merits in some circumstances, there appears a trend toward a more flexible and easy-to-access way of cognitive remediation, and these preliminary results seemed encouraging with regard to feasibility and patient satisfaction.

Concerning the impact of cognitive rehabilitation for POMS, these studies also showed promising results. More or less improvements in targeted cognitive domains were reported in all three studies, although discrepancy was noted between subjective and objective measures [23]. Given the heterogeneity and limited number of studies and their small sample size, no recommendation can be made for specific type of cognitive rehabilitation for POMS. It is noteworthy that the study on attention training showed far transfer effect [24], which is plausible because different facets of cognition could affect one another. These cross-modal effects deserve more exploration in future studies. Two studies of cognitive rehabilitation included neuroimaging evaluation [22,23], and one of them found correlation between working memory network activation and behavioral response [22], providing preliminary evidence that functional training is viable. Admittedly, more research is needed to resolve the controversial issue of functional training versus strategy training in cognitive rehabilitation for pediatric MS [42,43]. Sophisticated neuroimaging techniques may help to answer this question, as well as to clarify whether and how neuroplastic changes are facilitated by rehabilitation [44].

This scoping review has some limitations. First, we do not address social cognition, which appears more dissociable from other aspects of cognition and requires a separate approach [45,46]. Second, we do not examine studies of exercise training and its cognitive effects in pediatric patients with MS. There have been suggestions that physical activity may exert beneficial effects on cognition for both youth and MS patients, although more research in this direction is needed [47–49]. Third, given that our focus is on the cognitive assessment tools, we do not include studies aiming to characterize the cognitive profile of POMS. Nonetheless, we should acknowledge that in a broad sense many of those studies also contributed supportive evidence for the validity of various assessment tools.

5. Conclusions

Experiences with cognitive assessment tools for POMS are accumulating. Nonetheless, more research into their psychometric properties along the disease course may aid in the selection of appropriate tools during different disease stages. Computer-administered cognitive assessment and rehabilitation may be a trend worthy of further investigation. Systematic studies with larger sample size and rigorous methodology are much needed to inform evidence-based cognitive rehabilitation for POMS.

Supplementary Materials: The following are available online at http://www.mdpi.com/2227-9067/7/10/183/s1, Supplementary File S1: PRISMA-ScR Checklist, Supplementary File S2: Scoping Review Protocol.

Author Contributions: Conception and design of the study: W.-S.L. and S.-J.L.; acquisition and analysis of data: W.-S.L., S.-J.L., T.-R.H.; preparation of tables and figures: W.-S.L. and S.-J.L.; drafting the manuscript: W.-S.L.; critical review of the manuscript for intellectual content: W.-S.L., S.-J.L., T.-R.H. All authors have read and agreed to the published version of the manuscript.

Funding: This research received no external funding.

Conflicts of Interest: The authors declare no conflict of interest.

References

1. Waldman, A.; Ness, J.; Pohl, D.; Simone, I.L.; Anlar, B.; Amato, M.P.; Ghezzi, A. Pediatric multiple sclerosis: Clinical features and outcome. *Neurology* **2016**, *87*, S74–S81. [CrossRef] [PubMed]
2. Carotenuto, A.; Moccia, M.; Costabile, T.; Signoriello, E.; Paolicelli, D.; Simone, M.; Lus, G.; Brescia Morra, V.; Lanzillo, R. Associations between cognitive impairment at onset and disability accrual in young people with multiple sclerosis. *Sci. Rep.* **2019**, *9*, 18074. [CrossRef] [PubMed]
3. Wallach, A.I.; Waltz, M.; Casper, T.C.; Aaen, G.; Belman, A.; Benson, L.; Chitnis, T.; Gorman, M.; Graves, J.; Harris, Y.; et al. Cognitive processing speed in pediatric-onset multiple sclerosis: Baseline characteristics of impairment and prediction of decline. *Mult. Scler.* **2019**. [CrossRef] [PubMed]
4. Julian, L.; Serafin, D.; Charvet, L.; Ackerson, J.; Benedict, R.; Braaten, E.; Brown, T.; O'Donnell, E.; Parrish, J.; Preston, T.; et al. Cognitive impairment occurs in children and adolescents with multiple sclerosis: Results from a United States network. *J. Child Neurol.* **2013**, *28*, 102–107. [CrossRef]
5. Johnen, A.; Elpers, C.; Riepl, E.; Landmeyer, N.C.; Kramer, J.; Polzer, P.; Lohmann, H.; Omran, H.; Wiendl, H.; Gobel, K.; et al. Early effective treatment may protect from cognitive decline in paediatric multiple sclerosis. *Eur. J. Paediatr. Neurol.* **2019**, *23*, 783–791. [CrossRef]
6. Wuerfel, E.; Weddige, A.; Hagmayer, Y.; Jacob, R.; Wedekind, L.; Stark, W.; Gartner, J. Cognitive deficits including executive functioning in relation to clinical parameters in paediatric MS patients. *PLoS ONE* **2018**, *13*, e0194873. [CrossRef]
7. Brenton, J.N.; Koshiya, H.; Woolbright, E.; Goldman, M.D. The Multiple Sclerosis Functional Composite and Symbol Digit Modalities Test as outcome measures in pediatric multiple sclerosis. *Mult. Scler. J. Exp. Transl. Clin.* **2019**, *5*, 2055217319846141. [CrossRef]
8. Kapanci, T.; Rostasy, K.; Hausler, M.G.; Geis, T.; Schimmel, M.; Elpers, C.; Kreth, J.H.; Thiels, C.; Troche, S.J. Evaluating the relationship between psychometric intelligence and cognitive functions in paediatric multiple sclerosis. *Mult. Scler. J. Exp. Transl. Clin.* **2019**, *5*, 2055217319894365. [CrossRef]
9. Amato, M.P.; Goretti, B.; Ghezzi, A.; Hakiki, B.; Niccolai, C.; Lori, S.; Moiola, L.; Falautano, M.; Viterbo, R.G.; Patti, F.; et al. Neuropsychological features in childhood and juvenile multiple sclerosis: Five-year follow-up. *Neurology* **2014**, *83*, 1432–1438. [CrossRef]
10. Charvet, L.E.; O'Donnell, E.H.; Belman, A.L.; Chitnis, T.; Ness, J.M.; Parrish, J.; Patterson, M.; Rodriguez, M.; Waubant, E.; Weinstock-Guttman, B.; et al. Longitudinal evaluation of cognitive functioning in pediatric multiple sclerosis: Report from the US Pediatric Multiple Sclerosis Network. *Mult. Scler.* **2014**, *20*, 1502–1510. [CrossRef]
11. Arksey, H.; O'Malley, L. Scoping studies: Towards a methodological framework. *Int. J. Soc. Res. Methodol.* **2005**, *8*, 19–32. [CrossRef]
12. Tricco, A.C.; Lillie, E.; Zarin, W.; O'Brien, K.K.; Colquhoun, H.; Levac, D.; Moher, D.; Peters, M.D.J.; Horsley, T.; Weeks, L.; et al. PRISMA Extension for Scoping Reviews (PRISMA-ScR): Checklist and Explanation. *Ann. Intern Med.* **2018**, *169*, 467–473. [CrossRef] [PubMed]
13. Portaccio, E.; Goretti, B.; Lori, S.; Zipoli, V.; Centorrino, S.; Ghezzi, A.; Patti, F.; Bianchi, V.; Comi, G.; Trojano, M.; et al. The brief neuropsychological battery for children: A screening tool for cognitive impairment in childhood and juvenile multiple sclerosis. *Mult. Scler.* **2009**, *15*, 620–626. [CrossRef] [PubMed]
14. Falco, F.; Moccia, M.; Chiodi, A.; Carotenuto, A.; D'Amelio, A.; Rosa, L.; Piscopo, K.; Falco, A.; Costabile, T.; Lauro, F.; et al. Normative values of the Rao's Brief Repeatable Battery in an Italian young adolescent population: The influence of age, gender, and education. *Neurol. Sci.* **2019**, *40*, 713–717. [CrossRef]
15. Smerbeck, A.M.; Parrish, J.; Yeh, E.A.; Hoogs, M.; Krupp, L.B.; Weinstock-Guttman, B.; Benedict, R.H. Regression-based pediatric norms for the brief visuospatial memory test: Revised and the symbol digit modalities test. *Clin. Neuropsychol.* **2011**, *25*, 402–412. [CrossRef] [PubMed]
16. Smerbeck, A.M.; Parrish, J.; Yeh, E.A.; Weinstock-Guttman, B.; Hoogs, M.; Serafin, D.; Krupp, L.; Benedict, R.H. Regression-based norms improve the sensitivity of the National MS Society Consensus Neuropsychological Battery for Pediatric Multiple Sclerosis (NBPMS). *Clin. Neuropsychol.* **2012**, *26*, 985–1002. [CrossRef] [PubMed]
17. Bigi, S.; Marrie, R.A.; Till, C.; Yeh, E.A.; Akbar, N.; Feinstein, A.; Banwell, B.L. The computer-based Symbol Digit Modalities Test: Establishing age-expected performance in healthy controls and evaluation of pediatric MS patients. *Neurol. Sci.* **2017**, *38*, 635–642. [CrossRef]

18. Charvet, L.E.; Beekman, R.; Amadiume, N.; Belman, A.L.; Krupp, L.B. The Symbol Digit Modalities Test is an effective cognitive screen in pediatric onset multiple sclerosis (MS). *J. Neurol. Sci.* **2014**, *341*, 79–84. [CrossRef]
19. Charvet, L.E.; Shaw, M.; Frontario, A.; Langdon, D.; Krupp, L.B. Cognitive impairment in pediatric-onset multiple sclerosis is detected by the Brief International Cognitive Assessment for Multiple Sclerosis and computerized cognitive testing. *Mult. Scler.* **2018**, *24*, 512–519. [CrossRef]
20. Smerbeck, A.M.; Parrish, J.; Serafin, D.; Yeh, E.A.; Weinstock-Guttman, B.; Hoogs, M.; Krupp, L.B.; Benedict, R.H. Visual-cognitive processing deficits in pediatric multiple sclerosis. *Mult. Scler.* **2011**, *17*, 449–456. [CrossRef]
21. Storm Van's Gravesande, K.; Calabrese, P.; Blaschek, A.; Rostasy, K.; Huppke, P.; Rothe, L.; Mall, V.; Kessler, J.; Kalbe, E. The Multiple Sclerosis Inventory of Cognition for Adolescents (MUSICADO): A brief screening instrument to assess cognitive dysfunction, fatigue and loss of health-related quality of life in pediatric-onset multiple sclerosis. *Eur. J. Paediatr. Neurol.* **2019**, *23*, 792–800. [CrossRef] [PubMed]
22. Hubacher, M.; DeLuca, J.; Weber, P.; Steinlin, M.; Kappos, L.; Opwis, K.; Penner, I.K. Cognitive rehabilitation of working memory in juvenile multiple sclerosis-effects on cognitive functioning, functional MRI and network related connectivity. *Restor. Neurol. Neurosci.* **2015**, *33*, 713–725. [CrossRef] [PubMed]
23. Till, C.; Kuni, B.; De Somma, E.; Yeh, E.A.; Banwell, B. A feasibility study of working memory training for individuals with paediatric-onset multiple sclerosis. *Neuropsychol. Rehabil.* **2019**, *29*, 1177–1192. [CrossRef] [PubMed]
24. Simone, M.; Viterbo, R.G.; Margari, L.; Iaffaldano, P. Computer-assisted rehabilitation of attention in pediatric multiple sclerosis and ADHD patients: A pilot trial. *BMC Neurol.* **2018**, *18*, 82. [CrossRef] [PubMed]
25. Brandstadter, R.; Katz Sand, I.; Sumowski, J.F. Beyond rehabilitation: A prevention model of reserve and brain maintenance in multiple sclerosis. *Mult. Scler.* **2019**, *25*, 1372–1378. [CrossRef] [PubMed]
26. Kalb, R.; Beier, M.; Benedict, R.H.; Charvet, L.; Costello, K.; Feinstein, A.; Gingold, J.; Goverover, Y.; Halper, J.; Harris, C.; et al. Recommendations for cognitive screening and management in multiple sclerosis care. *Mult. Scler.* **2018**, *24*, 1665–1680. [CrossRef] [PubMed]
27. Margoni, M.; Rinaldi, F.; Riccardi, A.; Franciotta, S.; Perini, P.; Gallo, P. No evidence of disease activity including cognition (NEDA-3 plus) in naive pediatric multiple sclerosis patients treated with natalizumab. *J. Neurol.* **2020**, *267*, 100–105. [CrossRef]
28. Duignan, S.; Brownlee, W.; Wassmer, E.; Hemingway, C.; Lim, M.; Ciccarelli, O.; Hacohen, Y. Paediatric multiple sclerosis: A new era in diagnosis and treatment. *Dev. Med. Child Neurol.* **2019**, *61*, 1039–1049. [CrossRef]
29. Amato, M.P.; Morra, V.B.; Falautano, M.; Ghezzi, A.; Goretti, B.; Patti, F.; Riccardi, A.; Mattioli, F. Cognitive assessment in multiple sclerosis-an Italian consensus. *Neurol. Sci.* **2018**, *39*, 1317–1324. [CrossRef]
30. Amato, M.P.; Goretti, B.; Ghezzi, A.; Lori, S.; Zipoli, V.; Portaccio, E.; Moiola, L.; Falautano, M.; De Caro, M.F.; Lopez, M.; et al. Cognitive and psychosocial features of childhood and juvenile MS. *Neurology* **2008**, *70*, 1891–1897. [CrossRef]
31. Bartlett, E.; Shaw, M.; Schwarz, C.; Feinberg, C.; DeLorenzo, C.; Krupp, L.B.; Charvet, L.E. Brief Computer-Based Information Processing Measures are Linked to White Matter Integrity in Pediatric-Onset Multiple Sclerosis. *J. Neuroimaging* **2019**, *29*, 140–150. [CrossRef] [PubMed]
32. Amato, M.P.; Goretti, B.; Ghezzi, A.; Lori, S.; Zipoli, V.; Moiola, L.; Falautano, M.; De Caro, M.F.; Viterbo, R.; Patti, F.; et al. Cognitive and psychosocial features in childhood and juvenile MS: Two-year follow-up. *Neurology* **2010**, *75*, 1134–1140. [CrossRef] [PubMed]
33. Benedict, R.H.; Amato, M.P.; Boringa, J.; Brochet, B.; Foley, F.; Fredrikson, S.; Hamalainen, P.; Hartung, H.; Krupp, L.; Penner, I.; et al. Brief International Cognitive Assessment for MS (BICAMS): International standards for validation. *BMC Neurol.* **2012**, *12*, 55. [CrossRef] [PubMed]
34. Filser, M.; Schreiber, H.; Pottgen, J.; Ullrich, S.; Lang, M.; Penner, I.K. The Brief International Cognitive Assessment in Multiple Sclerosis (BICAMS): Results from the German validation study. *J. Neurol.* **2018**, *265*, 2587–2593. [CrossRef]
35. Toussaint-Duyster, L.C.; Wong, Y.Y.M.; Van der Cammen-van Zijp, M.H.; Van Pelt-Gravesteijn, D.; Catsman-Berrevoets, C.E.; Hintzen, R.Q.; Neuteboom, R.F. Fatigue and physical functioning in children with multiple sclerosis and acute disseminated encephalomyelitis. *Mult. Scler.* **2018**, *24*, 982–990. [CrossRef]
36. Amato, M.P.; Krupp, L.B.; Charvet, L.E.; Penner, I.; Till, C. Pediatric multiple sclerosis: Cognition and mood. *Neurology* **2016**, *87*, S82–S87. [CrossRef]

37. MacAllister, W.S.; Christodoulou, C.; Troxell, R.; Milazzo, M.; Block, P.; Preston, T.E.; Bender, H.A.; Belman, A.; Krupp, L.B. Fatigue and quality of life in pediatric multiple sclerosis. *Mult. Scler.* **2009**, *15*, 1502–1508. [CrossRef]
38. Aaen, G.; Waltz, M.; Vargas, W.; Makhani, N.; Ness, J.; Harris, Y.; Casper, T.C.; Benson, L.; Candee, M.; Chitnis, T.; et al. Acquisition of Early Developmental Milestones and Need for Special Education Services in Pediatric Multiple Sclerosis. *J. Child Neurol.* **2019**, *34*, 148–152. [CrossRef]
39. Mazerolle, E.L.; Wojtowicz, M.A.; Omisade, A.; Fisk, J.D. Intra-individual variability in information processing speed reflects white matter microstructure in multiple sclerosis. *Neuroimage Clin.* **2013**, *2*, 894–902. [CrossRef]
40. Harand, C.; Daniel, F.; Mondou, A.; Chevanne, D.; Creveuil, C.; Defer, G. Neuropsychological management of multiple sclerosis: Evaluation of a supervised and customized cognitive rehabilitation program for self-used at home (SEPIA): Protocol for a randomized controlled trial. *Trials* **2019**, *20*, 614. [CrossRef]
41. Nauta, I.M.; Speckens, A.E.M.; Kessels, R.P.C.; Geurts, J.J.G.; de Groot, V.; Uitdehaag, B.M.J.; Fasotti, L.; de Jong, B.A. Cognitive rehabilitation and mindfulness in multiple sclerosis (REMIND-MS): A study protocol for a randomised controlled trial. *BMC Neurol.* **2017**, *17*, 201. [CrossRef] [PubMed]
42. Hulst, H.E.; Langdon, D.W. Functional training is a senseless strategy in MS cognitive rehabilitation: Strategy training is the only useful approach—NO. *Mult. Scler.* **2017**, *23*, 930–932. [CrossRef] [PubMed]
43. Leavitt, V.M. Functional training is a senseless strategy in MS cognitive rehabilitation: Strategy training is the only useful approach—YES. *Mult. Scler.* **2017**, *23*, 928–929. [CrossRef] [PubMed]
44. Chiaravalloti, N.D.; Genova, H.M.; DeLuca, J. Cognitive rehabilitation in multiple sclerosis: The role of plasticity. *Front. Neurol.* **2015**, *6*, 67. [CrossRef] [PubMed]
45. Charvet, L.E.; Cleary, R.E.; Vazquez, K.; Belman, A.L.; Krupp, L.B. Social cognition in pediatric-onset multiple sclerosis (MS). *Mult. Scler.* **2014**, *20*, 1478–1484. [CrossRef] [PubMed]
46. Ekmekci, O. Pediatric Multiple Sclerosis and Cognition: A Review of Clinical, Neuropsychologic, and Neuroradiologic Features. *Behav. Neurol.* **2017**, *2017*, 1463570. [CrossRef] [PubMed]
47. Lubans, D.; Richards, J.; Hillman, C.; Faulkner, G.; Beauchamp, M.; Nilsson, M.; Kelly, P.; Smith, J.; Raine, L.; Biddle, S. Physical Activity for Cognitive and Mental Health in Youth: A Systematic Review of Mechanisms. *Pediatrics* **2016**, *138*. [CrossRef] [PubMed]
48. Yeh, E.A.; Kinnett-Hopkins, D.; Grover, S.A.; Motl, R.W. Physical activity and pediatric multiple sclerosis: Developing a research agenda. *Mult. Scler.* **2015**, *21*, 1618–1625. [CrossRef]
49. Sandroff, B.M.; Pilutti, L.A.; Benedict, R.H.; Motl, R.W. Association between physical fitness and cognitive function in multiple sclerosis: Does disability status matter? *Neurorehabil. Neural Repair* **2015**, *29*, 214–223. [CrossRef]

Publisher's Note: MDPI stays neutral with regard to jurisdictional claims in published maps and institutional affiliations.

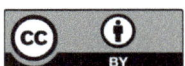

© 2020 by the authors. Licensee MDPI, Basel, Switzerland. This article is an open access article distributed under the terms and conditions of the Creative Commons Attribution (CC BY) license (http://creativecommons.org/licenses/by/4.0/).

MDPI
St. Alban-Anlage 66
4052 Basel
Switzerland
Tel. +41 61 683 77 34
Fax +41 61 302 89 18
www.mdpi.com

Children Editorial Office
E-mail: children@mdpi.com
www.mdpi.com/journal/children

www.ingramcontent.com/pod-product-compliance
Lightning Source LLC
LaVergne TN
LVHW070546100526
838202LV00012B/399